C10/79

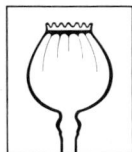

Current Topics in Anaesthesia

General Editors: Stanley A. Feldman
Cyril F. Scurr

4 Medical Problems and the Anaesthetist

Medical Problems and the Anaesthetist

Leon Kaufman, MD, FFA,RCS

Consultant Anaesthetist
University College Hospital, London and
St Mark's Hospital, London

and

Edward Sumner, MA, BM, BCh(Oxon), FFA,RCS

Consultant Anaesthetist
The Hospital for Sick Children, Great Ormond Street, London

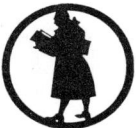

Edward Arnold

First published 1979
by Edward Arnold (Publishers) Ltd
41 Bedford Square, London WC1B 3DQ

British Library Cataloguing in Publication Data

Kaufman, Leon
  Medical problems and the anaesthetist.—(Current topics in anaesthesia; 4).
  1. Anaesthesia
  I. Title   II. Sumner, Edward   III. Series
  617'.96   RD81
  ISBN 0-7131-4341-X

Text set in 10/11 pt Monophoto Times and
printed in Great Britain by Butler & Tanner Ltd, Frome and London

General preface to series

The current rate of increase of scientific knowledge is such that it is recognized that '... ninety per cent of all the existing knowledge which can be drawn upon for the practice of medicine is less than 10 years old'.*

In an acute specialty, such as anaesthesia, failure to keep abreast of advances can seriously affect the standard of patient care. The need for continuing education is widely recognized and indeed it is mandatory in some countries.

However, due to the flood of new knowledge which grows in an exponential fashion greatly multiplying the pool of information every decade, the difficulty which presents itself is that of selecting and retrieving the information of immediate value and clinical relevance. This series has been produced in an effort to overcome this dilemma.

By producing a number of authoritative reviews the Current Topics Series has allowed the General Editors to select those in which it is felt there is a particular need for a digest of the large amount of literature, or for a clear statement of the relevance of new information.

By presenting these books in a concise form it should be possible to publish these reviews quickly. Careful selection of authors allows the presentation of mature clinical judgement on the relative importance of this new information.

The information will be clearly presented and, by emphasizing only key references and by avoiding an excess of specialist jargon, the books will, it is hoped, prove to be useful and succinct.

It has been our intention to avoid the difficulties of the large textbooks, with their inevitable prolonged gestation period, and to produce books with a wider appeal than the comprehensive, detailed, and highly specialized monographs. By this means we hope that the Current Topics in Anaesthesia Series will make a valuable contribution by meeting the demands of continuing education in anaesthesia.

Westminster Hospital London

Stanley A. Feldman
Cyril F. Scurr

*Education and Training for the Professions.
 Sir Frank Hartley, Wilkinson Lecture
 Delivered at Institute of Dental Surgery, 30.1.78
 University of London Bulletin, May 1978, No. 45, p. 3

Preface

This book is intended to supplement, and not replace, comprehensive text-books of medicine. It is concerned with the important medical hazards encountered when treating the surgical patient, especially in the preoperative preparation. The text concentrates on the medical background of the patient and the problems that arise during anaesthesia and surgery. Topics which are of particular importance or of special interest have been included, with each section giving an up-to-date review of the current literature. The text has been confined to considering the cardiovascular system, the respiratory system, haematology and endocrine organs.

All medical staff who are supervising the care of surgical patients will find the book particularly useful. Physicians, surgeons and anaesthetists who are involved in the preoperative preparation of surgical patients should find the information both stimulating and interesting. Candidates for the Final FFA,RCS examination and even their teachers will find important information assembled and collated from many sources.

Permission to publish figures 3.14–3.18 has been given by Dr T. D. Kellock, and the editor of the *Lancet*, whilst figures 3.5, 3.6, 3.7, 3.8, 3.10 on Phaeo-chromocytoma are reproduced by the permission of the editor of the *British Medical Journal*. It is our pleasure to acknowledge the assistance given to us by our faithful secretaries Enid Grattan-Guinnes and Elisabeth Moore.

London, 1979   L.K.
E.S.

Contents

1

Cardiovascular system

Cardiac and vascular pathology is common throughout all age groups and each presents its special problems. Cardiac pathology may, directly or indirectly, affect the function of all other organs, particularly the lungs, kidneys and brain. Potent drugs are administered to control hypertension, myocardial ischaemia with angina, arrhythmias and cardiac failure. Anaesthetic agents and techniques may have a profound direct or indirect action on cardiac function and tissue perfusion, and in addition may interact with the drugs already modifying myocardial function.

General anaesthesia often depresses myocardial function and predisposes to arrhythmias; although the arterial Po_2 and Pco_2 and pH are usually well maintained during anaesthesia, they may be temporarily upset during induction and recovery. The homoeostatic reflexes which normally make adjustments to loss of circulating blood volume, to posture and to fever are depressed by anaesthesia and narcotic agents.

The surgery itself imposes strains on the cardiovascular system, depending on the type of surgery, its site and extent. It also increases the risk of complications, which may include thromboembolic disease, renal and septic complications.

The cardiac index (cardiac output per square metre body surface area) of patients who survive major surgery rises and remains at elevated levels for several days postoperatively, whereas in patients who do not survive, there has been a low cardiac index preoperatively and has remained unaltered postoperatively (Perlroth and Hultgren, 1975).

Congenital heart disease

The incidence of congenital heart disease in the USA was shown by Richards *et al.* in 1955 to be 8·3 per 1000 total births (7·4 per 1000 live births), though the possible incidence may be 10 per 1000. The incidence appears to have remained constant and seems to be the same throughout the world.

If the patient is undiagnosed, congenital heart disease should be suspected if cyanosis is present without an obvious respiratory cause. Congenital abnormalities are often multiple, and up to 20 per cent of cases have abnormalities

1

in other organs. Midline defects are often multiple; for example, ventricular septal defect (VSD), cleft palate and imperforate anus are seen together, and tracheo-oesophageal fistula is often combined with a cardiac defect. With the exception of the rubella syndrome, there is very little evidence to support any postulated extrinsic factors which might influence a developing fetus.

The older classification into cyanotic and acyanotic groups is unsatisfactory and classifications with embryological or anatomical bases are better. These include ventricular septal defects (VSD), atrial septal defect (ASD) (primum, secundum), abnormalities of the great vessels (transposition, truncus arteriosus), abnormalities of valves (pulmonary stenosis or atresia), patent ductus arteriosus, coarctation of the aorta, abnormalities of the great veins. The tetralogy of Fallot, the commonest of those conditions which cause cyanosis at rest (some 70 per cent of this group), consists of a VSD and pulmonary stenosis, often of the subvalvar type. The anatomy is rather variable and, depending on the size of the pulmonary arteries, may be difficult to correct fully. The over-riding of the aorta and the right ventricular hypertrophy (RVH) follow from the two main defects associated with this syndrome.

Congenital cardiac lesions are assuming a greater importance as more and more are being totally corrected with an ever-decreasing risk. Those very severe lesions for which there is no corrective operation are often amenable to palliative procedures which usually involve some anastomatic shunt between the systemic and pulmonary circulations. The significance is that, as these patients grow, they will from time to time need general surgical treatment, possibly away from the centre which dealt with their original cardiac defect.

Serious lesions in the newborn produce either severe hypoxia or cardiac failure, or both, and need urgent medical and surgical attention. Total anomalous pulmonary venous drainage and aortic stenosis are lesions for which immediate open heart surgery is necessary. A preductal coarctation must be resected as soon as the diagnosis is made and the severe hypoxia of pulmonary or tricuspid atresia must be relieved by a systemic–pulmonary shunt.

Other lesions may cause progressive problems; for example, VSD or single ventricle may cause pulmonary hypertension of an irreversible type. Pulmonary hypertension was thought to be rare under the age of 6 months but Haworth et al. (1977) have shown from post-mortem studies that there is impairment of growth and development of the pulmonary circulation dating from birth. Where the pulmonary artery pressure is equal to or higher than systemic, there occurs a narrowing of the external diameter of the small pulmonary arterioles, a reduction in the number of small intra-acinar vessels, an increase in the muscularity of the pulmonary arteries and an extension of muscularity to arteries not normally muscularized in infancy. In about half of these cases the pulmonary arterial (PA) pressure will fall after breathing 100 per cent oxygen. This would test the operability of the lesion because, if the PA pressure failed to fall and the change within the lung vasculature were irreversible, to close the VSD would be to precipitate fatal right ventricular failure. In patients under 4 years of age there is rarely evidence of the obliterative pulmonary vascular disease seen in older patients when the increased pulmonary vascular resistance becomes irreversible. This may progress to reverse the intracardiac shunt right to left and cause the progressive cyanosis of Eisenmenger's syndrome.

The VSD may cause serious changes in the pulmonary vasculature even from the very earliest age. Where the VSD has been closed early, the pulmonary vascular resistance remains high—although there is evidence that this eventually returns to normal.

The pathophysiological consequences of increasing pulmonary vascular disease are higher workload for the right ventricle and occasionally the right atrium, ventilation/perfusion abnormalities in the lungs with increased stiffness (decreased compliance), increased work of breathing and raised airway resistance.

An increased alveolar–arterial oxygen difference ($A-aDo_2$) may be manifest as cyanosis. As the situation deteriorates further, the left to right shunt will reverse; this gives the clinical picture of cyanosis, dyspnoea, haemoptysis, syncope, chest pain and progressive clubbing. If left to nature, the history of a severe VSD will be underdevelopment of the child and progressively severe episodes of cardiac failure in infancy. Then follows a period of relative fitness in the first and second decades of life, after which is seen a rapid downhill course when the shunt reverses (right to left). Death usually occurs with a syncopal attack in which there is a profound fall in the cardiac output as a result of sudden increased pulmonary vascular resistance.

With large shunts between the left and right sides of the heart, the size and direction of the shunt may be altered, and an increased right to left shunt can occur with an increase in pulmonary vascular resistance or a sudden fall in systemic blood pressure. The pulmonary vascular resistance can increase under the influence of hypoxia or CO_2 retention or decrease in pH. Sudden falls in systemic pressure may occur after induction of anaesthesia, with vasodilator drugs or following severe haemorrhage.

Patients with the Eisenmenger syndrome (high pulmonary vascular resistance and reversal of a shunt at aortopulmonary, atrial or ventricular level) withstand pregnancy poorly; in a series reported by Jones and Howitt (1965) there was a 30 per cent maternal mortality, which is much higher than that reported for other forms of congenital heart disease. The diagnosis of the syndrome is a contraindication to pregnancy, but the risk of termination of an established pregnancy carries just as high a risk as allowing it to continue. With great care, and delivery by caesarian section, successful outcome can be achieved. Falls in systemic blood pressure occur with induction of anaesthesia or positive pressure ventilation, and oxytocin decreases the total peripheral resistance.

In the puerperium when these patients first get out of bed, syncope may occur which is associated with a rise in pulmonary artery pressure. Similarly, during straining, the pulmonary artery pressure rises and thus increases the right to left shunt (Cutforth, Catchlove and Knight, 1968).

Tetralogy of Fallot

Among the problems associated with this lesion (before total correction or palliative shunting) are cyanosis and polycythaemia which predispose to thrombotic complications. Haemoglobin and the haematocrit are always monitored as a guide to progress before correction. During preparation for surgery, dehydration must be avoided and intravenous fluids must be given if starvation for more than 4 hours is contemplated. The contrast used for cardioangiography is an osmotic diuretic, and polycythaemic patients are at risk from cerebral thrombosis after this procedure unless intravenous fluids are given.

In addition, there may be disturbances of coagulation with reduced platelet function and increased fibrinolytic activity. These are found in most cases of cyanotic congenital heart disease.

Most of the blood is in the systemic circulation (venous hypertrophy) and there exists a delicate balance between the left and right circulation. If this is disturbed, the right to left shunt will increase. These patients need a high cardiac filling pressure and it is thought that the 'squatting' so characteristic of the Fallot patient is an attempt to help the filling pressure and to keep a high systemic peripheral resistance.

Changes in the right ventricular outflow tract obstruction can occur and are worsened particularly under the influence of β-adrenergic stimulation, pain, fear and isoprenaline. The increase in infundibular tone and spasm cause a reversal of the shunt, allowing 'hypercyanosis' and reduction of cardiac output. The infundibular spasm responds to morphine or β-adrenergic blockade. Isoprenaline is contraindicated. An increase in the systemic peripheral resistance helps to reverse the increased right to left shunt.

Unless an acidosis is progressive and severe, sodium bicarbonate should not be given. Most chronically cyanosed patients have a low serum bicarbonate (base excess -6) and have adjusted the oxygen dissociation curve to the right to compensate for this. To 'correct' this chronic, compensated state is a disservice to the patient in terms of oxygen delivery to the tissues. Severe acidosis should be corrected back to the compensated level.

Untreated cases of cyanotic congenital heart disease eventually die from hypoxia and its sequelae. One-third die from infection, often cerebral abscess which may start by infection in a small cerebral infarct. The cerebrovascular accidents which are a feature of advanced cyanotic heart disease are probably more often associated with relative anaemia than with a high haematocrit.

Arrhythmias

Spontaneous severe arrhythmias are uncommon in congenital heart disease, with the exception of the rare Ebstein's malformation which may be associated with the Wolff–Parkinson–White syndrome (see p. 13). The malformation involves downward displacement of the tricuspid valve, rendering it incompetent and causing the incorporation of the upper part of the right ventricle into the right atrium. The ventricular cavity is very small, with thin and flabby walls. Arrhythmias appear spontaneously associated with conduction disturbances, and the clinical picture is one of mild cyanosis, dyspnoea on exertion and congestive cardiac failure.

Prevention of bacterial endocarditis

Palmer and Kempf (1939) showed that *Streptococcus viridans* bacteraemia could follow dental extractions. They obtained positive blood cultures in 14 out of 82 patients. Patients with congenital heart disease, corrected or un-corrected (except secundum ASD), chronic valvular disease and cardiomyo-pathy are at risk of developing subacute bacterial endocarditis with such a bacteraemia. The risk of bacteraemia exists during any form of dental treatment but is highest if gingival bleeding is provoked. Genitourinary sur-gery also carries a high risk of bacteraemia.

Prevention of endocarditis with prophylactic antibiotics has been variable. A circular from dentists in Oxfordshire in 1975 showed that regimens were variable and only 12 per cent gave parenteral antibiotics (Leading article, 1977).

The American Heart Association recommendations are possibly those which should be followed (Kaplan *et al.*, 1977): preoperatively 1 MU benzyl-penicillin and 600 000 U procaine penicillin by intramuscular injection, fol-lowed by eight, 6-hourly doses of 500 mg penicillin V orally. For patients with prosthetic heart valves already having penicillin prophylaxis, 1 g of streptomycin is added to the preoperative injection.

For patients with a penicillin allergy, 1 g of vancomycin intravenously or a course of erythromycin, or both, is suggested. Separate regimens are pro-posed for patients needing genitourinary surgery, for which ampicillin and gentamicin are used against the predominantly Gram-negative organisms.

Anaesthesia

Though the effects of anaesthetic agents and techniques on myocardial func-tion and regional blood flow are discussed later, certain effects are peculiar to the patient with congenital heart disease.

A cardiologist's opinion is always of value, and any cardiac failure must be brought under control. A note must be made of medication (e.g. diuretics, β blockers, digoxin) and recent values of haemoglobin, packed cell volume (PCV) and electrolytes, especially K^+.

Normal premedication is well tolerated and anaesthesia should be con-ducted in a suitable environment with facilities for monitoring and resuscita-tion. The radial arteries should, where possible, be left intact for a corrective operation where this is pending. Of particular importance are the problems associated with pulmonary vascular disease, reversal of shunts and lung com-pliance changes secondary to a high pulmonary blood flow. Pulmonary vas-cular disease causes increased airways resistance by reducing airway calibre. Anaesthetic insults may include: an increase in A–aDo_2; a fall in cardiac out-put, in circulating blood volume, in arterial Po_2; a rise in arterial Pco_2; the induction of arrhythmias; and the increase in the work of breathing. Care must be taken to avoid upsetting the delicate balance which often exists in a left to right shunt situation. A vicious cycle of increasing systemic desaturation can be established because low arterial Po_2 causes reduced peripheral resistance but increases pulmonary vascular resistance.

During induction and maintenance of anaesthesia, care should be taken to prevent falls in systemic blood pressure—though not at the expense of peripheral vasoconstriction. Careful monitoring of the ECG and arterial pressure and a continuous clinical assessment of the peripheral circulation (warm, well perfused extremities) are essential, as is the need to maintain constant circulating blood volume and cardiac filling pressures. Central venous pressure monitoring in helpful. When the patient is polycythaemic, blood loss may be replaced with plasma. It is necessary to avoid the known factors associated with increasing pulmonary vascular resistance or infundibular spasm (e.g. hypoxia or hypercapnia and excessive intrathoracic pressure from intermittent positive pressure ventilation (IPPV). Spontaneous breathing anaesthetic techniques should probably be avoided except for very short surgical procedures.

It is said that agents provoking an increase in sympathetic activity, such as ether or cyclopropane, should be avoided; while it is true that increased β-adrenergic effects may be harmful in cases of the tetralogy of Fallot (and hypertrophic obstructive cardiomyopathy), the very fast and smooth induction of anaesthesia achieved with the use of cyclopropane outweighs any disadvantage.

Hypercyanotic attacks can be fatal, especially if associated with general anaesthesia. Acidosis must be carefully corrected (to base excess of -6 if the patient is already cyanosed) and measures taken to increase the systemic blood pressure by the administration of a pressor agent (e.g. methoxamine). Isoprenaline should be avoided because of its effect on the right ventricular outflow tract. The similar β-adrenergic stimulation from fear or light anaesthesia should also be avoided.

Postoperative ventilation and oxygenation must be maintained. Peripheral vasoconstriction may be a sign of increasing acidosis and a warning of less than optimal conditions. The use of mechanical ventilation per- and postoperatively should be considered much earlier for patients with limited cardiorespiratory reserve than for normal patients.

However, with careful monitoring and a suitable choice of anaesthetic technique, this type of patient can be handled with minimal cardiovascular disturbance.

Pulmonary hypertension and cor pulmonale

Chronic cor pulmonale is right ventricular hypertrophy resulting from disease affecting the function and/or structure of the lung except where these alterations are the result of conditions which primarily affect the left side of the heart or congenital heart disease (Thomas, 1972). Cor pulmonale is not equivalent to cardiac failure because ventricular hypertrophy ensues long before cardiac failure. The increased workload occurs because of vasoconstriction (reversible) or obliteration (irreversible) in the pulmonary vasculature, or both. The obstructive pulmonary hypertension seen in chronic bronchitis results from long-standing constriction of small pulmonary arteries which eventually become thickened. Permanent small artery lesions occur in sarcoidosis, pneumoconiosis and bronchiectasis, and can also follow thromboembolic disease. Right heart failure is a late stage and is always associated with severe pulmonary hypertension and hypoxia. The increased Pa_{CO_2} may lead to oedema because of renal retention of salt and water.

The normal pulmonary artery pressure (Ppa) at rest is less than 20 mmHg and there exists a significant relation between Ppa increase and reduction in forced expiratory volume in 1 second (FEV_1). Long-term oxygen breathing in chronic bronchitis gives a fall in Ppa by up to 10 per cent, possibly by regression of muscular hyperplasia of small pulmonary vessels. The fall is not maintained after the oxygen breathing stops, and thus these patients benefit from domiciliary controlled oxygen therapy (Abraham, Cole and Bishop, 1968). As the disability increases, the heart rate is raised relative to the oxygen uptake. Hypoxic pulmonary hypertension without infection leads to right ventricular hypertrophy, thickening of arteriolar walls and duplication of elastic laminae which is irreversible. Some of the increases in Ppa possibly result from hypoxia associated with chronic obstructive airways disease leading to increased vascular change. The subsequent ventilation/perfusion inequalities play a large part in making the patient hypoxic and thereby further increasing the vascular resistance. The stiff lungs increase the work of breathing and, as ventilation/perfusion inequalities deteriorate, further CO_2 retention occurs.

The site of stimulation for pulmonary vasoconstriction which causes the hypertension is not known; the precapillary segment, however, is known to be sensitive to an increase or decrease of H^+, possibly by interference with Na^+ and K^+ exchanges across smooth muscle membranes, leading to depolarization and increased action potentials.

Chronic respiratory failure leads to potassium depletion not well reflected in serum levels. The cardiac arrhythmias associated with pulmonary heart disease and the sensitivity to digitalis may possibly be explained by this depletion (Thomas and Valibhji, 1969).

Acute cor pulmonale is caused by acute or chronic respiratory failure in patients with generalized obstructive respiratory disease. All aspects of ventilatory function are impaired in these patients, and marked uncompensated respiratory acidosis shows that further CO_2 retention has occurred very recently.

Most patients with acute cor pulmonale have no evidence of right ventricular hypertrophy. The event which precipitates the condition is an added bronchitis or bronchopneumonia or even a severe and prolonged attack of bronchial asthma. A sudden increase in respiratory obstruction or reduction in alveolar ventilation will reduce blood oxygenation to dangerous levels. The controlling mechanisms of respiration in the central nervous system are susceptible to low oxygen saturation and a loss of ventilatory drive ensues. Hypoventilation is disastrous in these circumstances. The right ventricle fails as the pulmonary artery pressure rises to systemic levels with the increase in pulmonary vascular resistance caused partly by hypoxia but mainly by the mechanical effects in the lung of inflammatory reaction or air trapping. If the heart is already compromised by ischaemic disease and in the presence of hypoxia, congestive cardiac failure occurs when a marked rise in venous pressure is accompanied by a reduced cardiac output.

Controlled oxygen therapy must be initiated at once. Antibiotics and physiotherapy are needed, and antispasmodic drugs are often given though their effect in the very acute situation is not thought to be very valuable unless asthma is a contributory factor.

Digoxin and diuretics are necessary.

The combination of borderline or overt respiratory failure and cardiac failure must present the anaesthetist with his most difficult patient. Cardiac failure must be treated with digoxin and diuretics (and potassium replacement therapy); respiratory disease must be treated with antibiotics, antispasmodics and physiotherapy. Steroids and antibiotics are now used in most cases where asthma is a factor. For elective surgery attempts must be made to achieve a maximal state of fitness. Preoperative respiratory function testing and baseline blood gases are useful prognostically. The avoidance of excessive doses of respiratory depressant analgesics is essential. Postoperatively, the patient will need oxygen therapy with controlled inspired oxygen concentration and physiotherapy, and may need mechanical respiratory support (see Chapter 2).

References

Abraham, A. S., Cole, R. B. and Bishop, J. M. (1968). Reversal of pulmonary hypertension by prolonged oxygen administration to patients with chronic bronchitis. *Circulation Research* **23**, 147.

Cutforth, R., Catchlove, B. and Knight, L. W. (1968). Eisenmenger's syndrome and pregnancy. *Australian and New Zealand Journal of Surgery* **8**, 202.

Haworth, S. G., Sauer, U., Buhlmeyer, K. and Reid, L. (1977) The development of the pulmonary circulation in ventricular septal defect: a quantitative structural study. *American Journal of Cardiology* **40**, 781.

Jones, A. M. and Howitt, G. (1965). Eisenmenger's syndrome in pregnancy. *British Medical Journal* **2**, 1627.

Kaplan, E., Anthony, B. F., Bisno, A., Durack, D., Houser, H., Millard, D., Sanford, J., Schulman, S. T. *et al.* (1977). Committee Report, American Heart Association. *Circulation* **56**, 139A.

Leading article (1977). Prevention of endocarditis. *British Medical Journal* **4**, 1564.

Palmer, H. D. and Kempf, M. (1939). *Streptococcus viridans* bacteremia following extraction of teeth; case of multiple mycotic aneurysms in pulmonary arteries: report of cases and necropsies. *Journal of the American Medical Association* **113**, 1788.

Perlroth, M. G. and Hultgren, H. N. (1975). The cardiac patient and general surgery. *Journal of the American Medical Association* **232**, 1279.

Richards, M. R., Merritt, K. K., Samuels, M. M. and Longman, A. G. (1955). Congenital malformations of the cardiovascular system in a series of 6053 infants. *Pediatrics* **15,** 12.

Thomas, A. J. (1972). Chronic pulmonary heart disease. *British Heart Journal* **34,** 653.

Thomas, A. J. and Valibhji, P. (1969). Arrhythmias and tachycardia in pulmonary heart disease. *British Heart Journal* **31,** 491.

Myocardial infarction and the surgical patient

Operations on patients with recent coronary infarctions are known to be hazardous; the risks of reinfarction have been put as high as 100 per cent, and the mortality as high as 40 per cent. However, when two years have elapsed the risk may be no greater than with the rest of the population of the same age. Ischaemic heart disease affects about 20 per cent of the adult male population under 60 years of age.

A report from the Mayo Clinic has done a great deal to clarify the situation with regard to surgery in the patient with a recent coronary thrombosis (Tarhan *et al.*, 1972). In a series of 32 000 patients, the incidence of coronary thrombosis (using the normal diagnostic criteria, ECG, enzymes, etc.) in the first postoperative week was 20 times higher in patients with a history of a coronary infarction than in normal patients: 6·6 per cent compared with 0·13 per cent (in patients over 30 years of age). The mortality from these infarcts was 54 per cent (the same as in the group having the first infarction in the postoperative period). This mortality is very high compared with deaths in the coronary care units (20–30 per cent). It may be caused by additional factors associated with the surgery and anaesthesia, but may also be related to the fact that coronary care units do not usually see the patients who die immediately after the attack. The presence of refractory nocturnal or crescendo angina gives a risk of myocardial infarction as great as that after a recent coronary thrombosis.

Neither the duration nor the form of the anaesthesia appears to add to the risk, but the incidence of infarction increases in patients operated on for thoracic and upper abdominal conditions.

The liability to further infarction does not increase with age and it occurs most commonly during the third postoperative day.

Thus the risk of further infarction *is* increased but not to prohibitive levels except within three months of the first attack. Of patients operated on within three months, 37 per cent had postoperative reinfarction, 16 per cent operated on between three and six months and 4–5 per cent after six months.

Thus, after six months the risk of reinfarction is back to what it is in any patient after a previous attack—approximately 5 per cent.

Ischaemic heart disease has a high incidence of reinfarction and the anaesthetist should be aware of the factors which influence coronary arterial flow and the risks of surgery in patients with this disease.

Goldman *et al.* (1977) studied 1001 patients over 40 years of age scheduled for non-cardiac surgery and were able to identify nine independent correlates of life-threatening and fatal cardiac complications.

(1) Preoperative third heart sound or jugular venous distension.

(2) Myocardial infarction within the last six months.

(3) More than 5 premature ventricular contractions per minute documented at any time before operation.

(4) Rhythm; other than sinus, or the presence of premature atrial contractions on the preoperative ECG.

(5) Age; over 70 years.

(6) Intraperitoneal, intrathoracic or aortic operations.

(7) Emergency operations.

(8) Important valvular aortic stenosis.

(9) Poor general medical condition.

Coronary flow depends on perfusion pressure (diastolic pressure is the most important determinant), the resistance of small vessels and the degree of extravascular compression. These variables are determined by the rate of the heart, its contractility, the ventricular volume and pressure, and the left ventricular end-diastolic pressure (LVEDP). An increase in preload (increased filling pressure) or afterload (increased peripheral resistance) will raise the LVEDP, as does decreased myocardial contractility. In diastole an increase in LVEDP can mean myocardial ischaemia in the subendocardial layers, especially if the oxygenation is already prejudiced by ischaemic heart disease, or a hypertrophied ventricle. The resistance of small vessels is affected by drugs and both sympathetic and parasympathetic tone. The action of nitroglycerin in relieving angina is probably not by direct coronary vasodilatation but by the reduction in preload and afterload (Smith, 1976).

Anaesthetic drugs can have profound effects on the coronary circulation because of variations in oxygen demand rather than by direct action on the vessels. Halothane, it is claimed, reduces myocardial flow in all areas to a greater extent than the fall in metabolic activity. Myocardial tissue oxygenation may be improved more easily by reducing the oxygen demand rather than by increasing flow, as attempts to do this will increase the preload on the heart and impair the subendocardial circulation and oxygenation.

Optimal myocardial oxygenation is achieved by ensuring that the patient has a normal Hb level and haematocrit, that displacements of the oxygen dissociation curve to the left are avoided and that hypoxia and profound hypotension are prevented. Efforts should be made to maintain left ventricular volume and end-diastolic pressure as low as possible, by keeping a minimum preload and afterload, Arrhythmias will increase oxygen demands, as will increases in cardiac rate. Careful use of β blockers might be considered, as a reduction in sympathetic tone will help to reduce oxygen demands.

During surgery, monitoring should be as complete as possible using the ECG, direct or indirect blood pressure and central venous pressure readings. Blood gas analysis is also helpful although such monitoring is crude compared with, and gives little clue to what is happening to, intracardiac pressures and myocardial oxygen demands. Agents which stimulate β-

adrenergic activity (tachycardia and raised cardiac output) may be best avoided (e.g. cyclopropane, ether, gallamine and ketamine).

Arrhythmias (Dysrhythmia)

All arrhythmias reduce cardiac efficiency and tend to give a fixed, lower cardiac output. Atrial fibrillation is the commonest arrhythmia seen preoperatively but, as with all others, should be brought under control before surgery.

Those arrhythmias needing treatment are rare in well managed cases, though they may be interpreted as a warning of distress and that anaesthetic conditions are less than optimal. The ECG appearance gives no guide as to the effect on the circulation nor does it identify the mechanism responsible. The state of the circulation should be carefully monitored separately. Slow supraventricular rhythms need no treatment, but ventricular ones may be used as a sign of a more serious condition and should be treated as significant until proved otherwise (Katz and Bigger, 1970).

The incidence of arrhythmias varies and is governed by many factors. Arrhythmias are seen in 16·3 per cent of patients with no known heart disease, in 26·6 per cent of those with previous arrhythmias and in 34·4 per cent of those with previous heart disease. The overall incidence is 17·9 per cent. The commonest of 'induced' arrhythmias is the slow supraventricular rhythm but single nodal beats or runs of nodal beats and ventricular ectopics are all seen. They are less common in those below 30 years of age but occur more frequently if the patients are intubated; 20 per cent occur on induction although the incidence depends on the anaesthetic agents used. Of digitalized patients, 43 per cent have an arrhythmia some time during anaesthesia. However, only an estimated 0·9 per cent are serious, indicating that the heart is severely stressed, that the cardiac output has fallen and that surgical or anaesthetic conditions are not ideal. Most arrhythmias are explicable in terms of imbalance of the autonomic nervous system; however, they may be due not only to primary changes in the heart but also to primary changes in the central nervous system or in the periphery.

The reported incidence of arrhythmias increases if the ECG is written out rather than shown on a screen, but basically it is related to a very large number of possible factors associated with anaesthesia and surgery.

Spontaneously breathing patients show a higher incidence of arrhythmias than those with controlled ventilation. It has been suggested that thresholds of Pa_{CO_2} exist above which arrhythmias are seen, and that the thresholds differ according to the anaesthetic agent in use. In one series of animal experiments the threshold with cyclopropane occurred between 5·9 kPa and 9·6 kPa (44 and 72 mmHg) Pa_{CO_2} (mean 7·7 kPa or 58 mmHg) and with halothane in clinical doses between 8·0 kPa and 18·6 kPa (60 and 140 mmHg) (mean 12·3 kPa or 92 mmHg). The mechanism is thought to be catecholamine release via a brain stem reflex because stellate ganglion block abolishes these arrhythmias (Price et al., 1958).

Hypoxia also causes arrhythmias, both by a direct effect on the myocardium and indirectly via carotid and aortic chemoreceptors involving an increase in circulating catecholamines.

Large doses of catecholamines in the unanaesthetized patient can cause arrhythmias. The catecholamines can be exogenous or endogenous, or both. In the presence of cyclopropane or halogenated hydrocarbon anaesthetic agents, the dose of catecholamines needed to produce arrhythmias is very much reduced (as much as one-tenth of the previous dose). This is the so-called 'sensitization' of the myocardium. Very many cases of adrenergic-induced cardiac arrhythmias and cardiac arrest (ventricular fibrillation) in anaesthetized patients have been described in the literature. The arrhythmias are also more common, when serum potassium is raised, in the presence of a tachycardia or raised blood pressure, and if either a raised Pa_{CO_2} or a low Pa_{O_2} exists.

The arrhythmias caused by catecholamines may be blocked directly by β-adrenergic blockers and indirectly by α-adrenergic blockade (because of a fall in blood pressure). Beta blockers may also be effective because of their quinidine-like action.

When adrenaline (usually for local vasoconstrictive purposes) is to be injected into anaesthetized patients, Katz and Epstein (1968) have suggested that strengths of $1:100\,000$ to $1:200\,000$ should not be exceeded and that the total adult dose should not exceed 10 ml of $1:100\,000$ over 10 minutes or more than 30 ml per hour. These doses should be safe in the presence of halothane, trichloroethylene and other halogenated hydrocarbon anaesthetic agents. If there is a need for bronchiolar dilatation during anaesthesia, it is logical to use salbutamol, which has less β action on the heart.

Reflexes can initiate changes in the cardiac rate and rhythm; for example, the afferent limb coming from the larynx, pharynx, eye muscles and visceral structures. Various combinations of stimulation of the sympathetic or parasympathetic nervous systems are possible; tachycardias tend to be blocked by β blockers and bradycardias by atropine. Many are seen only with light anaesthesia. The oculocardiac reflex which occurs when the extraocular muscles are stretched (as in squint surgery) is largely abolished by atropine. However, if arrhythmias still occur they are said to be of a more serious type (more ventricular) and longer lasting.

The incidence of reflex arrhythmias associated with endotracheal intubation varies according to the series reported, ranging from 0 to 90 per cent. The incidence thus probably depends on many factors, particularly the anaesthetic agents being used at the time. An incidence of 50 per cent is quoted after intubation using deep halothane anaesthesia, but much less after thiopentone and relaxation using suxamethonium. The cause of intubation arrhythmias is not entirely understood; they are unimportant in a fit, well ventilated patient but may become significant and cause cardiac decompensation in those with incipient cardiac failure, cerebrovascular disease or phaeochromocytoma. They are largely mediated by the sympathetic nervous system, and the incidence can be reduced by β blockers and, to a great extent, by local anaesthesia of the respiratory tract.

The frequent occurrence of cardiac arrhythmias in association with dental anaesthesia is very well documented and is seen in up to 34 per cent of cases in reported series (Ryder and Townsend, 1974). The types of change in rhythm range from supraventricular to functional and ventricular. The arrhythmias are not necessarily associated with extractions, though most occur at this time; up to half were seen before the extraction actually began. Most of the ECG changes are benign, though in the presence of halogenated hydrocarbon anaesthetic agents more ventricular ectopics are seen; these latter are probably more significant in patients with pre-existing cardiac disease. The incidence is reduced by β blockers and also if the reflex arc is broken by a local anaesthetic block before the teeth are extracted. Certainly where there is pre-existing cardiac disease or an arrhythmia is present, it is sensible to use local anaesthesia when practicable in addition to general anaesthesia. For major dental work, dental clearances, etc., in the cardiac patient, a technique using controlled ventilation and local anaesthesia is recommended. Local anaesthesia without sedation may be more harmful than general anaesthesia itself because of the emotional stress and increased endogenous catecholamines induced in frightened, awake patients. Those with aortic or mitral stenosis are prone to sudden attacks of pulmonary oedema or even sudden death, especially if a change in cardiac rhythm is provoked by anaesthesia.

The effects of the changes and imbalance of electrolytes, particularly potassium, on arrhythmias are important. Hypokalaemia leads to an increased rate of diastolic depolarization, giving an increased rate of discharge of automatic membranes and a production of ectopic rhythms. Hypokalaemia must be the most common cause of changes in cardiac rhythm associated with cardiac surgery, cardiopulmonary bypass and large doses of diuretics (associated with metabolic alkalosis). Potassium may safely be given intravenously at a concentration not exceeding 4 mmol in 100 ml if the ECG is monitored carefully during the infusion.

Possibly associated with an increase in serum potassium are the severe ventricular arrhythmias seen when suxamethonium is used in patients with renal failure. This potassium shift has been shown to occur particularly in patients with burns, massive trauma, spinal cord injury and hemiplegia (Galindo and Davies, 1962). After an injection of suxamethonium the serum potassium level rises approximately 0·5 mmol/litre and may disturb the seemingly crucial ratio of intracellular to extracellular potassium. Suxamethonium should be avoided in burned patients (two to seven weeks after the burns is the period of highest risk) and in patients with renal failure. There are many reports of cardiac arrest associated with the use of suxamethonium in these circumstances, but there are also reports of arrhythmias with its use in normal patients. Bradycardia, sinus arrest, supraventricular and ventricular arrhythmias are seen, especially after a second dose of the drug. It has been suggested that choline, a product of the hydrolysis of suxamethonium, sensitizes the patient to succinylcholine. Pretreatment with thiopentone seems to reduce this sensitization and atropine prevents it. These cardiovascular actions of suxamethonium may be blocked by β blockers or ganglion blockade. Bradycardias are prevented by atropinization of the patient, though atropine itself can cause arrhythmias.

The Wolff–Parkinson–White syndrome (described in 1930) has ECG changes of a short P–R interval (0·12 s or less), a wide QRS complex as seen in bundle branch block (0·11 s or more), a δ wave and a history of tachy-cardias. It is caused by abnormal anatomical tracts which bypass the atrio-ventricular (AV) node, thus making a re-entrant loop and causing 'pre-excita-tion' of the ventricle. The usual abnormality is an anterograde AV nodal and retrograde bypass conduction. In childhood three-quarters of the patients suffer from spontaneous paroxysmal tachycardia which can be very difficult to treat, though procainamide is effective in some cases (Mandel and Laks, 1975). Twelve per cent are associated with other congenital heart defects. Other treatment consists of atrial pacing with increasing rates until anterograde conduction block occurs. The maximum rates which can be used are those at which AV conduction is still 1:1. The patients usually live out normal lives, though the effect of the arrhythmias is worsened in later life with the development of coronary artery disease. Anaesthesia with its poss-ible insults of hypoxia, hypercarbia, and reduced cardiac output, and those factors which put the oxygenation of the subendocardial layers at risk, may provoke attacks of paroxysmal tachyarrhythmias.

Most changes in cardiac rhythm need no treatment. Their presence should be noted and steps taken to eliminate any obvious causal factors. Occasion-ally, arrhythmias become intractable and may cause falls in cardiac output which must be reversed. These effects are always worse in the presence of pre-existing cardiac disease.

Bradycardias are effectively treated by intravenous atropine, except those caused by partial or complete AV dissociation. However, a tachycardia may have a deleterious effect on an ischaemic myocardium. Isoprenaline infusion (1 mg in 100 ml 5 per cent dextrose) at a rate of 1–3 μg per minute may be helpful for a bradycardia with AV block. Severe bradycardia should be treated by pacing or by external cardiac massage until pacing can be organized.

Supraventricular tachycardia may respond to carotid sinus massage (Chamberlain and Williams, 1976).

Digitalis is the drug of choice for supraventricular arrhythmias but is itself a common cause of arrhythmias in overdosage, especially when the serum potassium is low (hence the use of potassium supplements with diuretics). Digoxin may be given intravenously in a full digitalizing dose (1·5 mg) though fast atrial rates may not slow for some hours. A synchronized d.c. shock may be an alternative way of bringing down a very rapid rate, especially if the tachycardia is causing a low cardiac output. The primary therapeutic action of digitalis in the treatment of supraventricular tachyarrhythmias is to slow the ventricular rate by depressing atrioventricular conduction. Thus, types of AV block are the commonest manifestation of digoxin toxicity. If quinidine is to be used in the treatment of arrhythmias, it is important to remember that this drug can cause neuromuscular depression and may predispose to respiratory arrest. Disturbances of ventricular rhythm will not respond to carotid sinus massage.

Lignocaine, 1 mg/kg i.v., controls most ventricular arrhythmias and repeated doses or an infusion may be necessary. Beta blockers (e.g. proprano-lol, 1 mg i.v. over several minutes and repeated up to four times) may control tachycardias. Usually an effect is seen within 10 minutes though the use of

β blockers is inadvisable in the presence of serious myocardial dysfunction. D.C. shock may be necessary if the tachycardia does not respond to drug therapy before excessive and depressant doses have been given. D.C. shock is contraindicated where the arrhythmia is thought to be caused by digoxin overdose.

Other drugs to consider for refractory cases of tachyarrhythmias include disopyramide 150 mg i.v. over 10 minutes, or procainamide 100 mg i.v. every 5 minutes to a maximum of six to eight doses.

Ventricular fibrillation should be treated by d.c. defibrillation (200 joules) as soon as the diagnosis is made. If the principal cause is hypoxia, attempts must be made to reverse this state first. If the ventricular fibrillation is of very recent onset, mechanical defibrillation with a large thump on the precordium may be successful. Failing these, external cardiac massage and pulmonary ventilation with 100 per cent oxygen must be instituted. If the diagnosis is delayed, defibrillation is likely to be unsuccessful without first correcting the hypoxia and acidosis (1 mmol HCO_3/kg body weight initially). Attempts should be made to convert fine ventricular fibrillation to coarse ventricular fibrillation with the use of 10 per cent calcium chloride solution and 1 : 10 000 adrenaline by intravenous or intracardiac injection. After successful defibrillation, lignocaine infusion may be necessary, though this has no part in the treatment of the initial stages of cardiac arrest.

References

Chamberlain, D. A. and Williams, J. M. (1976). Immediate care of cardiac emergencies. *Anaesthesia* **31,** 760.

Galindo, A. H. and Davis, T. V. (1962). Succinylcholine and cardiac excitability. *Anesthesiology* **23,** 32.

Goldman, L., Caldera, D. L., Nussbaum, S. R., Southwick, F. S., Krogstad, D., Murray, B. *et al.* (1977). Multifactorial index of cardiac risk in noncardiac surgical procedures. *New England Journal of Medicine* **297,** 845.

Katz, R. L. and Bigger, J. T. (1970). Cardiac arrhythmias during anesthesia and operation. *Anesthesiology* **33,** 193.

Katz, R. L. and Epstein, R. A. (1968). The interaction of anesthetic agents and adrenergic drugs to produce cardiac arrhythmias. *Anesthesiology* **29,** 763.

Mandel, W. J. and Laks, M. M. (1975). Wolff–Parkinson–White syndrome: pharmacological effects of procainamide. *American Heart Journal* **90,** 744.

Price, H. L., Lurie, A. A., Jones, R. E., Price, M. L. and Linde, M. W. (1958). Cyclopropane anesthesia: epinephrine and norepinephrine in initiation of ventricular arrhythmias by carbon dioxide inhalation. *Anesthesiology* **19,** 619.

Ryder, W. and Townsend, D. (1974). Cardiac rhythm and dental anaesthesia. *British Journal of Anaesthesia* **46,** 760.

Smith, G. (1976). The coronary circulation and anaesthesia. (Editorial) *British Journal of Anaesthesia* **48,** 933.

Tarhan, S., Moffitt, E. A., Taylor, W. F. and Guiliani, E. R. (1972). Myocardial infarction after general anesthesia. *Journal of the American Medical Association* **220,** 1451.

Hypertension

Hypertension, treated or untreated, is the commonest abnormality of the cardiovascular system. The frequency of raised blood pressure seen in surgical patients of all ages has been estimated to be as high as 10–12 per cent and 1·4 per cent of all patients. The line between normotensive and hypertensive levels of blood pressure is drawn arbitrarily and depends on, among other things, the standard of living of the particular country. Life insurance statistics show that, over certain levels, life expectancy is reduced. Hypertension has been defined as 'that blood pressure above which investigation and treatment do more good than harm'.

Today, the patient with high blood pressure is subjected not only to the whole range of surgical procedures, but also to operations which are designed to correct the underlying cause of the hypertension.

There is little agreement about what constitutes normal blood pressure, and levels as great as 180/110 mmHg have been suggested as normal for advancing age. Often blood pressures are falsely raised when measured after admission to hospital and inaccuracies associated with the relation between the size of the upper arm and the width of the sphygmomanometer cuff may give false readings. Cuff size should be two-thirds of the length of the upper arm.

The finding of a raised pressure is only one sign of what may be a generalized disease, and it may be necessary to find a possible cause for the hypertension before a surgical procedure is undertaken. The effects of the hypertension itself must also be assessed by further tests. ECG and chest X-ray are mandatory and some tests of renal function, urine and serum electrolytes are the minimum that should be done before routine surgery in the hypertensive patient.

There is also an association between raised blood pressure and obesity, independent of difficulties in measurement associated with the large arm circumference. Mortality rates from coronary artery disease in obese hypertensives are higher than those for patients with either obesity alone or hypertension alone. It should be considered to be in the patient's interest for him to undergo a period of weight reduction before routine surgery.

Elderly hypertensives also show progressive falls in pulmonary function with increasing maldistribution of ventilation/perfusion and progressive airways closure, though this is usually less significant than the effects of the hypertension on the cardiovascular system.

The condition adds to the risk of both surgery and anaesthesia, and although the prognosis is improved if the blood pressure is controlled pharmacologically, the drugs themselves may interact with those used in anaesthesia and again the risks are increased. Life expectancy of patients with hypertension is inversely proportional to the increase in systolic and diastolic pressures.

One classification of hypertension is by degree; for example, as follows.

(1) Accelerated course, usually seen in the younger age groups and often has an identifiable cause. Such patients often have renal disease as a primary or secondary problem. If this hypertension is untreated, patients die in renal or cardiac failure or with cerebrovascular accidents.

(2) Benign course, usually essential hypertension.

Untreated hypertension in men increases the overall mortality tenfold, and in women eightfold. Myocardial infarction and angina are twice as frequent in hypertensives as in the rest of the population. The prognosis for pre-existing cardiac disease is worsened in the presence of hypertension. The longer the existence of hypertension, the more likely will be the presence of arteriosclerosis.

Hypertension is caused either by an increase in cardiac output by the mechanism of increased cardiac rate, myocardial contractility and increased ventricular filling pressure, or by increased peripheral resistance. This latter is usually the main component and is associated with a decrease in the cross-sectional area of the arteriolar bed, the vessel length or an increase in blood viscosity. The capillary bed becomes less able to convert pulsatile flow to more continuous flow.

The hypertension associated with renal artery stenosis is related to both types. The afterload on the left ventricle increases, leading to left ventricular hypertrophy, and the myocardial oxygen consumption increases more than necessary for the extra work involved.

The cause of essential hypertension is still a matter for conjecture (Hickler and Vandam, 1970). There is no good evidence of excess sympathetic activity leading to increased peripheral resistance. High serum sodium may be associated with hypertension and a low serum sodium may improve it, but there is no evidence that this defect is a primary causative factor of essential hypertension. Nor is there any real evidence of increased activity of the renin–angiotensin–aldosterone system as the aetiological basis of essential hypertension. In fact, the peripheral plasma renin activity is below normal in 20 per cent of cases and another subgroup shows abnormal aldosterone secretion in response to stimulation of the renin–angiotensin system. When hypertension becomes malignant, there is a uniform tendency for renal renin secretion to increase rapidly, giving secondary hyperaldosteronism.

The endocrine causes of hypertension account for between 5 and 10 per cent of cases, and are important and interesting because they are potentially curable surgically (e.g. phaeochromocytoma). Most patients with Cushing's disease are hypertensive. In primary aldosteronism the effects are due to an increase in sodium reabsorption and potassium excretion under the influence of excess of aldosterone. The hypertension may result from an increase in peripheral resistance, either because of increased arteriolar tone or due to narrowing of the arteriolar lumen from oedema of the vessel wall. The hypokalaemia and alkalosis which comprise a marked feature of this syndrome may be the source of arrhythmias and possibly abnormal reactions after the use of muscle relaxants.

Renal artery stenosis may cause hypertension by an increase in renin secretion from the juxtaglomerular apparatus because of the impaired renal blood flow. A reduction of 75 per cent or more in the cross-sectional area of the renal artery is needed before there is any reduction in the renal blood flow. The increased renin secretion leads to a raised production of the pressor hormone, angiotensin. The increased renin secretion from the kidney probably results not from a direct fall in renal perfusion pressure, but from the reduction in the sodium load presented to the macula densa of the distal renal tubule. However, raised levels of renin from the kidney with arterial stenosis are still found postoperatively even when there has been a significant fall in the blood pressure. Thus, it is not at all clear why secondary aldosteronism is not always associated with renal vascular hypertension since angiotensin stimulates aldosterone secretion.

The treatment of hypertension markedly reduces the incidence of pathological sequelae and, thus, the morbidity and mortality.

Antihypertensives

Common antihypertensive agents in clinical use may be classified as follows (Foex and Prys-Roberts, 1974).

Those acting on the central nervous system

An example here is clonidine, which has a central sedative effect, and also reduces plasma renin activity and the urinary excretion of aldosterone and catecholamines. After withdrawal of this drug, a rebound phenomenon of raised blood pressure to very high levels is sometimes seen. This rise can be reversed using α-adrenergic receptor blocking drugs, such as phentolamine. Clonidine slows the heart, the reduction in rate being greatest when the blood pressure is lowest. The cardiac output falls mainly because of the reduction in heart rate but also because of some reduction in venous return. The hypotension and bradycardia result from a direct action by the drug on vasomotor centres in the brain stem.

Interrupting stimuli from the central nervous system to the periphery

(1) Ganglion blockade, which is rarely used because of the undesirable effects on other cholinergic sites. Trimetaphan (Arfonad) is used in anaesthesia for induced hypotension when required. This short-acting drug also causes release of histamine and is thus contraindicated in cases of asthma.

(2) Adrenergic transmission blockade (e.g. α-methyldopa).

(3) Adrenergic receptor blockade (α and β blockers)

(a) Alpha blockers. Tolazoline is useful particularly to reverse the pulmonary vascular spasm causing persistent fetal circulation in babies.

Phentolamine is a short-acting α-blocking drug used for its systemic effect.

(b) Beta blockers (e.g. propranolol). The mechanism by which this drug causes a reduction in blood pressure is not entirely understood. The onset of action takes two to three weeks. There is a central action with a reduction in anxiety and in myocardial performance (possibly a quinidine-like action). In addition, there is inhibition of renin secretion and readjustment of baroreceptor reflexes, possibly because of the lowering of the renin–angiotensin system which may also reduce the peripheral resistance.

Decreased sensitivity of vascular smooth muscle

E.g. Hydrallazine, sodium nitroprusside and diazoxide. Diazoxide is related to the benzothiazidine diuretics but causes sodium retention.

Diuretics

All diuretic drugs act to reduce the plasma and extracellular volumes.

Thus, the antihypertensive drugs affect the central and peripheral autonomic nervous systems and also the end organs. In the past, it was the practice to discontinue these drugs before surgery in the hope that it would be better to have a patient with an intact homoeostatic mechanism for the maintenance of cardiac output and organ perfusion. Often this needed up to three weeks for the effects of certain drugs (e.g. α-methyldopa) to wear off, during which time the patients were again at risk from the effects of raised blood pressure. Recent opinion suggests that the drugs should be maintained until the day of the operation because of the risks of cardiovascular or cerebrovascular accident if the drugs are stopped and the blood pressure allowed to rise. Most anaesthetists regard the drug-treated hypertensive as a better anaesthetic risk. In the past the drugs were stopped because of the high incidence of bradycardia and hypotension occurring during anaesthesia in the presence of early hypotensive agents such as reserpine.

However, the hypertensive patient can have wide fluctuations in blood pressure even if untreated and the risk of vascular accident is such that starting drug treatment of the hypertension preoperatively is often to be recommended. The problems of the patients are related much more to the association of hypertension with ischaemic heart disease and cerebrovascular disease than to interactions between hypotensive drugs and anaesthetic agents.

Knowledge of which drug is involved and the pathological processes of the disease allows a choice of an appropriate anaesthetic technique, and the pharmacological action of the hypotensive drug suggests the correct pressor drug to be used (direct or indirect) if severe hypotension develops.

Several drugs have rebound effects if withdrawn; for example, clonidine. Wilson et al. (1969) showed that when a placebo was substituted for oxprenolol in a double-blind trial, 6 out of 18 patients suffered a severe increase in attacks of angina. Myocardial infarction may be causally related to abrupt withdrawal of propranolol, though this is difficult to prove because β blockers are used in the treatment of angina. In a trial of propranolol and a placebo in 20 patients with stable angina, and confirmed coronary artery disease, all the patients were well for 12 weeks' treatment with 160–320 mg daily doses of propranolol (Miller *et al.*, 1975). After propranolol was withdrawn and a placebo substituted, 2 patients died, 1 suffered ventricular tachycardia needing d.c. shock and 3 suffered a severe resurgence of angina at rest within 14 days; 4 others increased by more than 50 per cent their rate of attacks of angina. In the other 10 there was no change in the angina after withdrawal of propranolol, but in these patients there had been no great response when the drug was started in the first place. Thus, patients with myocardial disease treated with moderate doses of propranolol are at risk of important ischaemic complications if the drug is suddenly withdrawn, especially if the symptoms were markedly improved by the drug. Withdrawal must be followed by an increase in sympathetic drive to the heart and increased myocardial oxygen requirements.

Anaesthesia and hypertension

During anaesthesia all attempts must be made to maintain the circulatory state in optimal condition. The treated hypertensive suffers no greater fall in blood pressure during anaesthesia than the normal patient.

The patient with essential hypertension is often more agitated than the normal, and sedative needs are often greater.

Although the blood pressure as measured at the arm is not necessarily a good guide to organ blood flow, the blood pressure should not be allowed to fall to low levels. A low blood pressure will reduce coronary flow to various parts of the myocardium. Common causes of hypotension include overdosage of anaesthetic agents. Thiopentone for induction must be given slowly and in minimal quantities. Maintenance anaesthesia with halothane or other halogenated hydrocarbon anaesthetic agents for long periods may cause a fall in blood pressure.

Passive hyperventilation and hypocapnia lead to a decrease in ventricular stroke volume without changes in the cardiac rate or the mean blood pressure (Foex and Prys-Roberts, 1975). This is a direct CO_2 effect and is accompanied by an increase in systemic vascular resistance. In the absence of any significant increase in left ventricular end-diastolic pressure (LVEDP), the decrease in stroke volume can be accounted for by an increase in systemic vascular resistance. An acute rise in systemic vascular resistance may increase the systemic blood pressure but cause a decrease in stroke volume; this is seen in patients with poor left ventricular function and in patients after cardiopulmonary bypass. This reduction in ventricular stroke volume with hypocapnia caused by the inability of the ventricular muscle to maintain its ejection characteristics if depressed by anaesthetic agents (e.g. halothane) in the face of increasing systemic vascular resistance, occurs very frequently in the hypertensive patient. Where possible, normoventilation should be employed. Other causes of hypotension are hypovolaemia, traction reflexes occurring during inadequate planes of anaesthesia, mechanical interference with the venous return to the heart and, not uncommonly in the sick patient, a repeat myocardial infarction. The appearance of arrhythmia will cause a fall in blood pressure and cardiac output. The commonest arrhythmia is a junctional rhythm; this interferes with the contribution of the atria to ventricular filling at slow heart rates and can lead to a fall in cardiac output. Atropine does not consistently reverse this, but it can minimize the detrimental effect of this arrhythmia on atrial function. A decrease in perfusion pressure in elderly patients with cerebrovascular disease may lead to transient or permanent neurological damage. Patients with a previous stroke have a high risk of a second one during a hypotensive episode. Pressor amines are rarely needed if anaesthetic doses are judged correctly but should be used if the systemic pressure is falling to levels which are thought to be prejudicing myocardial blood flow. The action of these drugs is modified by antihypertensive therapy.

Pressor amines excite α-adrenergic receptors of vascular smooth muscle. Some do this direct (e.g. adrenaline or noradrenaline), whereas others act indirectly and cause the release of the natural sympathetic neurohumoral transmitter (e.g. methylamphetamine). Methoxamine probably has direct and indirect actions.

Ganglion and sympathetic blockers enhance the response to both the direct-acting and the normally occurring catecholamines. Drugs which deplete the stores of catecholamines in nerve endings, such as bethanidine, reserpine or α-methyldopa, reduce the efficiency of indirectly acting but enhance the action of directly acting pressor amines. Monoamine oxidase inhibitors lead to increased stores and thus there is a great over-reaction with the indirect types of vasopressor drug.

After the suitable drug has been chosen, it is advisable to make a dilution of one ampoule either in 10 ml in a syringe or in 100 ml in a microdrop burette and to give the drug very slowly in very small increments until the desired effect is reached. An overdose of vasopressor which causes a swing to the hypertensive state may be more harmful than the hypotension it is to correct.

Equally to be avoided is a hypertensive crisis during anaesthesia. Hypertensive crises occur in the presence of phaeochromocytoma and in patients taking monoamine-oxidase-inhibiting drugs when exposed to naturally occurring amines. They occur during eclampsia, in the malignant phase of hypertension and in acute or end-stage renal failure. In modern 'balanced' anaesthesia the depth of anaesthesia may be insufficient to block afferent impulses from the operative field (associated with increases in cardiac rate and rises in blood pressure). Cyclopropane and ether stimulate the sympathetic nervous system, and injected adrenaline for local vasoconstriction will also raise the blood pressure. Overload of the circulation by intravenous fluids should be avoided.

In the hypertensive patient, it is probable that an increase in blood pressure poses more of a threat to coronary perfusion than dose a fall in blood pressure, unless this is catastrophic. As the pressure rises, myocardial work is increased and there may not be an equal increase in the blood flow to all areas of the myocardium. Complete cessation of the subendocardial collateral blood supply may occur with a left ventricular end-diastolic pressure as low as 15–20 mmHg. This can easily occur with increases in the preload but more especially with the afterload of the ventricle caused by an increase in the systemic vascular resistance. As the subendocardial blood flow slows or ceases, the ECG patterns show ischaemia and ventricular extrasystoles are provoked.

A hypertensive crisis may be difficult to control. The depth of anaesthesia should be increased and positive pressure in the airway will cause a fall in the venous return to the heart and, hence, a fall in its output. Blood will pool in the periphery if the patient is placed in the reverse Trendelenburg position. If the hypertension is caused at least partly by peripheral vasoconstriction, drugs to reverse this may be used.

Chlorpromazine in increments of 2·5 mg intravenously is often very effective in reducing systemic blood pressure without causing much central sedation postoperatively. Care must be taken to give small doses incrementally or the fall in pressure may be profound. The central venous pressure may also fall and it may be necessary to give fluids intravenously to maintain central filling pressures. The α-blocking drug, phentolamine, in small increments intravenously is also effective in these circumstances, but is short acting. An infusion of sodium nitroprusside, with its direct effect on the vascular smooth muscle, is also recommended. This latter drug is being used increasingly to prevent excessive afterload on a left ventricle which is prejudiced either by ischaemic heart disease or after cardiopulmonary bypass. Its very prolonged use, or an increased dose in the face of resistance of action, or in very small babies is unwise. The usual dose is 5–10 ml per hour of a mixture of 50 mg in 500 ml of 5 per cent dextrose. For small children, the concentration may have to be increased, or transfused volumes of clear fluid will be excessive.

In hypertension the maintenance of systemic blood flow depends on the contractile state of the hypertrophied myocardium in the face of a constantly elevated peripheral vascular resistance. The response to anaesthesia must depend on the overall effect of the agent on the vascular resistance and myocardial contractility. *In vitro*, there is usually a dose-related depressant effect on myocardial function. At minimal alveolar concentration 1 (MAC 1) depression is seen with all anaesthetic agents, including cyclopropane, ether, enflurane, methoxyflurane and halothane. A mycocardium which is already hypertrophied is even more sensitive. In the intact patient there will be some compensation for this depression from the positive inotropic action of the sympathetic nervous system, but this varies according to which anaesthetic agent is used.

Anaesthetic requirements may also be modified by agents interfering with the sympathetic nervous system. A correlation has been shown between anaesthetic requirements and the concentration of noradrenaline in the central nervous system (Miller, Way and Eger, 1968). Thus the MAC of halothane is reduced by pretreatment with reserpine and α-methyldopa.

Anaesthetic effects on the circulation

All the potent general anaesthetic agents reduce myocardial contractile force in *in vitro* specimens, but cyclopropane (and ether, to a lesser extent) in the intact animal can, by virtue of stimulation of sympathetic nervous system, allow maintenance of cardiac output, a raised peripheral vascular resistance and an increase in venous return to the heart. Though this agent might seem to be the logical choice for use in the patient with hypertension, to maintain normal organ perfusion, the vascular homoeostasis is achieved at the expense of increased cardiac work, a rise in systemic pressure, and a heightened ventricular irritability. The increased secretion of catecholamines seen with cyclopropane anaesthesia causes a progressive decrease in the circulating blood volume, which may partly explain the postoperative hypotension sometimes seen after use of this agent. The central venous pressure rises as peripheral vasoconstriction occurs, thus increasing both preload and afterload for the left ventricle. The vasoconstriction is mediated in part by increased sympathetic tone and by increased responsiveness to and prolongation of the action of endogenous noradrenaline.

General anaesthesia causes a marked antidiuresis and a reduction in the glomerular filtration rate and renal plasma flow by about 50 per cent. This is mainly caused by a reduction in perfusion pressure but also by intrarenal vasoconstriction because of pain or trauma. Cyclopropane has a greater ischaemic effect on the activation of the renin–angiotensin system. Most anaesthetic agents diminish the effective splanchnic blood flow; cyclopropane by sympathetically mediated vasoconstriction and halothane by a general lowering of the perfusion pressure. In the hypertensive patient this could be harmful to the already marginally perfused liver. Halothane probably causes less reduction in hepatic blood flow than other agents and might thus be considered the agent of choice where borderline liver function is present. This agent would not, of course, be used in patients with a history of jaundice following previous halothane anaesthesia.

Halothane causes a fall in mean arterial pressure from a combination of reduction in cardiac output and a decrease in the peripheral resistance, but without much change in the venous distensibility. The sum effect may mean less work for the heart. In the early phases of halothane anaesthesia the blood flow to the periphery increases as the vessels dilate, and this state of a lower peripheral resistance with a slight fall in cardiac output may seem an ideal one. However, as anaesthesia proceeds, patients become increasingly vasoconstricted peripherally, perhaps reflexly as the cardiac output gradually falls.

Anaesthesia and heart disease

When anaesthesia is to be given to any patient with pre-existing heart disease, it is recommended that the following questions be posed (Foex, 1978): will the operation and associated anaesthesia overtax the heart and cause it to fail; does the heart need treatment preoperatively; is the cardiac prognosis so bad that the operation needs to be put off or limited to a palliative procedure; is the cardiac condition likely to lead to sudden death under anaesthesia?

Digoxin (together with diuretics) should be given to patients with congestive cardiac failure. However, the prophylactic use of digoxin does not prevent postoperative congestive cardiac failure and may increase the risk of overdosage and the therapy of arrhythmias postoperatively. The effects of digoxin overdose are worsened in the presence of hypokalaemia. Rapid digitalization therapy by the intravenous route is not without danger. The peripheral vasoconstrictor action of digitalis may precede the positive inotropic effect by an interval long enough to allow cardiac decompensation with right ventricular failure from an increase in ventricular afterload and increased myocardial oxygen demands which cannot be met.

Bradycardias from second degree heart block need preoperative pacemakers but, unless the patients have unexplained syncope, those with bundle branch block or first degree heart block do not need pacemakers. Demand pacemakers are sensitive to diathermy and should be converted to a fixed rate using a precordial magnet before surgery.

Severe angina may warrant coronary vein grafting surgery under cardiopulmonary bypass before elective general surgery is undertaken. The same applies to patients with cardiac decompensation with valvular disease. Arrhythmias must be diagnosed and treated accordingly, as must hypertension. Antibiotic prophylaxis against subacute bacterial endocarditis must be given to all patients with valve disease, cardiomyopathy and congenital heart disease except the secundum ASD (see p. 5).

Beta blockers are commonly used in patients with hypertension, hypertrophic obstructive cardiomyopathy, ischaemic heart disease, and, occasionally, in cases of tetralogy of Fallot. They must not be withdrawn preoperatively unless there is a very good indication; they are not now withdrawn before cardiopulmonary bypass because it takes at least 24 hours for the effects to wear off, in which time the patients are at risk of myocardial infarction. The drugs also reduce myocardial oxygen consumption during bypass, which is advantageous if aortic cross-clamping is used. If inotropic agents are needed after bypass, perhaps dopamine would be the drug of choice. Patients on β blockers may need intravenous atropine during anaesthesia as hypertensive patients are especially prone to bradycardia in the presence of β blockers or ganglion blockers. Patients on propranolol do not show different haemodynamic values (cardiac output, blood pressure and pulse rate) during anaesthesia from those without this drug (Kopriva, Brown and Pappas, 1978). They do not become hypertensive during intubation, and ECG signs of ischaemia are absent when hypocapnia is induced by passive hyperventilation. Haemodynamic values during acute haemorrhage are similar in β-blocked and non-blocked animals, as are the responses to short periods of hypoxia. Thus, on balance, the advantages are favourable for those patients with β blockade. However, β-blocked patients do not exhibit a tachycardia with hypovolaemia under general anaesthesia and the cardiac output will fall if β blockers are introduced when the output is maintained by the positive inotropic effect of sympathetic activity. Hypocapnia and hypoxia, which can develop peroperatively and at any time postoperatively, may depress the heart in the presence of β-blocking agents much more than in the normal patient. This is directly comparable with the situation whereby cardiac output is maintained by α-adrenergic activity and phentolamine or chlorpromazine are given.

Anaesthetic agents and techniques should be chosen for minimal cardio-vascular disturbances. Premedication should be adequate to minimize anxiety, as this might precipitate an attack of angina, but not so deep that respiratory or cardiovascular depression ensues. No induction agent is entirely satisfactory, though ketamine is unsuitable because of its tendency to increase hypertension and cardiac output. Intubation can cause arrhythmias and increases in blood pressure which can be avoided by local anaesthetic spray (or careful use of β blockers).

Patients undergoing operations on the lower abdomen, perineum or legs may be well managed with caudal, low spinal or epidural anaesthesia. High epidural anaesthesia interferes with vasomotor tone and often precipitates hypotension, and blockage of the sympathetic supply to the heart will reduce cardiac output. Light sedation in addition to a local anaesthetic procedure will reduce anxiety.

Deep planes of general anaesthesia should be avoided because they cause myocardial depression and a fall in coronary perfusion pressure, but a light plane of anaesthesia which just obtunds the sympathetic responses (manifesting themselves as sweating, tachycardia and increase in pulse rate) is desirable (Lappas, Powell and Doggett, 1977).

Monitoring for the patient at risk with cardiac disease must include the ECG and arterial blood pressure measurements. For major cases a cannula is placed percutaneously in one radial artery and this is feasible even in neonates. If the patient is to have corrective cardiac surgery in the near future, it is probably unwise to use a radial artery as these will be needed on that occasion. Arterial cannulation carries a low morbidity if some assessment is made of the peripheral circulation in the hand via the ulnar artery. Systemic pressure must be maintained within 15 per cent of the normal resting value for the patient, though not at the expense of reduced peripheral blood flow. The presence of a strong radial pulse in a warm, pink hand is a very reassuring sign. The peroperative causes of hypotension have been discussed earlier; they may include anaesthetic overdosage, hypovolaemia, manipulation of the heart or arrhythmias. The aim should be to restore coronary blood flow with as small an increase in oxygen consumption as possible and to keep the periphery well perfused. Urine flow may be used as a guide to adequacy of peripheral circulation and a minimum flow of 0·5 ml/kg body weight per hour should be sought. Dopamine in doses between 5 and 10 μg/kg per minute exerts a positive inotropic effect on the myocardium without greatly increasing its oxygen consumption. So specific is this myocardial effect that the receptors in the cardiac muscle have been called 'dopaminergic' receptors. Dopamine also specifically increases renal blood flow in moderate doses and thus maintains urinary output. In doses over 10μg/kg per minute, an α-adrenergic effect appears and becomes predominant as the dose is further increased.

Postoperatively, hypoxia must be prevented. Extubation and a stormy recovery from anaesthesia or postoperative shivering always carry a risk of hypoxia unless an increased inspired oxygen concentration is provided. All parameters of cardiac function should be monitored as closely as is necessary. With due care and with knowledge of the pathophysiological changes which occur as the result of cardiac disease, the anaesthetist can help to make more safe surgical procedures carried out on patients with pre-existing cardiac disease.

Cardiomyopathy

Cardiomyopathies are disorders of the heart muscle of unknown aetiology as opposed to those causes of cardiac muscular disease associated with an underlying disease; for example, haemochromatosis.

The latest and most satisfactory classification is based on the functional pathology (Goodwin, 1973):

(1) *Hypertrophic* with impaired diastolic compliance, with or without outflow tract obstruction.

(2) *Congestive* with poor systolic function.

(3) *Obliterative* endomyocardial fibrosis producing obliteration of the ventricular cavities.

The coronary artery supply is normal.

Hypertrophic obstructive cardiomyopathy (HOCM)

Hypertrophy of the ventricular septum and left ventricular outflow tract obstruction are usually the outstanding features, though obstruction may not be seen. There is a great decrease in the elasticity of the ventricular muscle and diastolic failure with filling difficulty. The magnitude of the LVEDP marks the extent of the involvement and is the main determinant of the severity of the symptoms and prognosis. The left ventricle fills slowly because of the non-pliant chamber and a tachycardia shortens diastolic filling time, leading to pulmonary oedema and syncope.

Surgical treatment involving incision and/or resection of the hypertrophied septum by various techniques does relieve symptoms. The surgery reduces the gradient and the accompanying mitral regurgitation, and decreases the LVEDP. Surgery is not indicated if obstruction is not present. The survival period does not seem to be extended after surgical relief of the obstruction.

The disease involves the whole myocardium and the LVEDP may increase again when the demands of exercise are made on the ventricle.

β-adrenergic stimulation (e.g. with inotropic agents (isoprenaline), exercise, pain or fear) increases the systolic outflow tract gradient. It was originally thought that the left ventricle became hyperkinetic with excess sympathetic activity, and an increase of adrenergic tissue in the outflow tract has been described. For these reasons and because there does seem to be an abnormal response to sympathetic stimulation, trials of β-adrenergic-blocking therapy were started on patients with cardiomyopathy. With treatment, the outflow tract obstruction is reduced, though the resting effect may be small. Beta blockade prevents an increase in outflow tract obstruction with isoprenaline. The incidence of angina is reduced, exercise tolerance is increased and there is a lowered incidence of syncope.

However, the incidence of sudden death does not seem to be lessened. Beta blockade is more effective when the outflow tract obstruction is latent or variable than if it is present at rest. Syncope and sudden death follow episodes of tachycardia. The increased heart rate leads to greater curtailment of left ventricular filling, a fall in stroke volume and blood pressure to a level where coronary flow becomes inadequate for myocardial oxygenation.

The progression of the disease is seen when the murmur disappears, congestive cardiac failure and atrial fibrillation follow. Left ventricular filling is further reduced by the atrial fibrillation. Anticoagulants should be given as thromboembolism is a risk. Digitalis should be used to control the ventricular rate because there is no outflow tract obstruction at this stage. Subacute bacterial endocarditis is a risk and antibiotics should always cover any surgery where bacteraemia is possible (dental and genitourinary surgery).

Congestive cardiomyopathy

Congestive cardiomyopathy allows only incomplete systolic ejection, leading to a dilated flabby heart. All other causes of left ventricular failure and constrictive pericarditis must be excluded before the diagnosis can be made. The clinical picture is of congestive cardiac failure, cardiomegaly and gallop rhythm; 10–15 per cent of patients have systemic hypertension.

The pathogenesis is not known. It is not more frequent in Jamaicans, as was once thought; 10 per cent of patients have angina and need coronary angiography for the diagnosis to be made. A small percentage have a history of previous myocarditis (e.g. infection by Coxsackie B virus). Alcoholism has been incriminated, and other possible causes are cobalt salts used as froth stabilizers in the brewing industry, thiamine deficiency or an as yet unproven direct effect which could possibly lower the resistance of the myocardium to other toxic agents. Certain cases seen in the peripartum period may be associated with multiparity and malnutrition. No genetic causes have been recognized.

Treatment consists of bed rest, digitalis and diuretics. Pericardiectomy may allow the fibres to work at a more favourable length–tension relation. There is no evidence of fundamental or long-lasting benefit to be gained from steroid therapy, though this is invaluable in rare specific cases of myocardial disease (e.g. sarcoidosis) so it is vital that these be diagnosed correctly.

Obliterative cardiomyopathy

The obliterative type of cardiomyopathy is very rare in the UK and no effective treatment is known.

Undiagnosed cases, especially of HOCM, are likely to give trouble during anaesthesia, where sudden death may follow a tachycardia; there are several reports of sudden death in these circumstances. Where anaesthesia is needed for diagnosed cases, halothane is best avoided and careful use made of β blockers to prevent tachycardia. Anaesthesia and monitoring should be conducted on the lines recommended for use in any patient with cardiac disease.

References

Foex, P. and Prys-Roberts, C. (1974). Anaesthesia and the hypertensive patient. *British Journal of Anaesthesia* **46**, 575.

Foex, P. and Prys-Roberts, C. (1975). Effect of CO_2 on myocardial contractility and aortic impedance during anaesthesia. *British Journal of Anaesthesia* **47**, 669.

Foex, P. (1978). Preoperative assessment of patients with cardiac disease. *British Journal of Anaesthesia* **50**, 15.

Goodwin, J. F. (1973). Treatment of the cardiomyopathies. *American Journal of Cardiology* **32**, 341.

Hickler, R. B. and Vandam, L. D. (1970). Hypertension. *Anesthesiology* **33**, 214.

Kopriva, C. J., Brown, A. C. D. and Pappas, G. (1978). Hemodynamics during anesthesia in patients receiving propranolol. *Anesthesiology* **48**, 28.

Lappas, D. G., Powell, W. M. J. and Doggett, W. M. (1977). Cardiac dysfunction in the peri-operative period. *Anesthesiology* **29**, 1153.

Miller, R. D., Way, W. L. and Eger, E. I. II (1968). The effects of alphamethyldopa, reserpine, guanethidine and iproniazid on minimum alveolar anaesthetic requirement (MAC). *Anesthesiology* **29**, 1153.

Miller, R. R., Olson, H. G., Amsterdam, E. A. and Mason, D. T. (1975). Propranolol-withdrawal/rebound phenomenon. *New England Journal of Medicine* **293**, 416.

Wilson, D. F., Watson, O. F., Peel, J. S. and Turner, A. S. (1969). Trasicor in angina pectoris: a double-blind trial. *British Medical Journal* **2**, 155.

2

Respiratory disease

All anaesthetists face the problem of patients with respiratory disease who need surgery. Pulmonary pathology is common in all age groups, though advancing age is a prime factor in the increase in pathology and subsequent postoperative complications. Postoperative pulmonary complications constitute 13–25 per cent of postoperative deaths and the incidence of such complications does not seem to be falling. Lung pathology affects anaesthesia, its uptake and distribution, and anaesthesia and surgery cause changes in ventilation/perfusion characteristics and airway closure in the lungs. A knowledge of the pathophysiology of chronic and acute lung disease is essential for the anaesthetist so he may minimize anaesthetic and surgical insults to the lung and to tissue oxygenation.

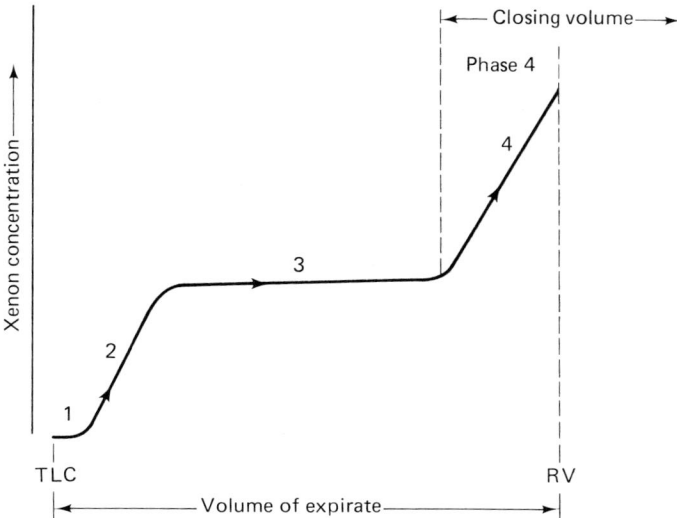

Fig. 2.1 The single breath technique for measurement of closing volume.

29

The concept of airway closure is very useful to explain changes which occur with age, with lung pathology and during anaesthesia (Craig *et al.*, 1971). At total lung capacity (TLC) all alveoli are evenly inflated; as lung volume decreases, however, dependent alveoli decrease in size more than those uppermost and, at some stage of lung deflation, airways begin to close. The lung volume at which airway closure starts is the closing volume (CV). When a patient is standing, airway closure occurs at the base of the lungs because of the effect of gravity; alveoli at the bases are stretched less and are therefore less well supported and more apt to close. Either loss of elastic recoil or airway instability can lead to an increase in CV, and in the absence of abnormal recoil an increase in CV shows small airways disease. CV may be measured by the single breath xenon method (Fig. 2.1). Normally CV is small and at a value close to the residual volume (RV) of the lung. During normal tidal ventilation at functional residual capacity (FRC) all dependent airways are open. (The Fowler curve has four phases; the junction between the third and fourth, at which the nitrogen concentration increases abruptly toward end-expiration, is when airway closure begins.) Thus the difference between FRC and CV should have a positive value. But CV can increase because of less elastic recoil or increased collapsibility of small airways, and can even encroach upon the end-tidal position and so small airways will be closed during normal breathing. As the blood supply to the bases is intact, this will be an area perfused but not ventilated, thus increasing an intrapulmonary R–L shunt and increasing $A–aDo_2$. In childhood and again with advancing age airways begin to close above FRC and the situation is made worse if the subject moves from the erect to the supine position. The diaphragm ascends and the subject then breathes at lower lung volumes for tidal breathing and more airways close during the breathing cycle.

During anaesthesia the relationship of FRC to CV (which is crucial for gas exchange) may change. Because measurements of CV need active help from the subject, they are difficult to make during anaesthesia; it is known, however, that FRC may be reduced during anaesthesia, compared with values taken before induction (Don, Wahba and Cuadrado, 1970). Stone *et al.* (1975) suggest that FRC may not increase during anaesthesia in healthy young patients so that it remains above CV throughout the respiratory cycle. Shunting should perhaps not be considered a normal phenomenon. The decrease in FRC is accompanied by an increase in the volume of trapped gas though the volume of the latter decreases as anaesthesia proceeds, suggesting it is progressively absorbed. The use of high concentrations of nitrogen during anaesthesia will not protect against the trapping and absorption of gas. Intermittent 'sighs' make no difference to either FRC or volume of trapped gas (Don, Wahba and Craig, 1972). The crucial factor in gas trapping is the relation between FRC and CV. When CV is increased as it is in the very young, the elderly, in the supine position or in the obese, and FRC is reduced as it is during anaesthesia, airway closure will occur during tidal breathing and gas will be trapped, the functional effect of which is impairment of gas exchange and increase in $A–aDo_2$. There is no progressive decrease in FRC as anaesthesia proceeds, neither does the shunt progressively increase (Nunn and Panday, 1968).

The concept of CV is also useful to explain the effects of constant distending pressure which, when used with intermittent positive airway pressure ventilation, is known as positive end-expiratory pressure (PEEP) and, with spontaneous ventilation, as constant positive airway pressure (CPAP). The ability of a constant distending pressure to raise arterial oxygenation with a constant inspired oxygen concentration depends on the relation between FRC and CV in the lungs. The effect of CV exceeding FRC and of right to left intrapulmonary shunting occurring is seen in disease states of the lung (e.g. pulmonary oedema, hyperperfused lungs). With the application of a constant distending pressure alveoli in the mid-regions of the lungs are opened (those in the non-dependent parts are already maximally taking part in ventilation). FRC increases in relation to CV with a reduction in the intrapulmonary shunt and a decrease in A–aDo$_2$ (Craig *et al.*, 1972).

Pulmonary function testing
(Fletcher *et al.*, 1963; Cotes, 1968; Hatch and Milner, 1974; Clarke, 1976)

Forced expiratory volume in 1 second (FEV$_1$) (or 0·75 s) and forced vital capacity (FVC) using the vitalograph comprise the basis of the simplest lung function tests. A great deal can be learned from the absolute figures and the ratio in terms of obstructive or restrictive chest lesions. Peak inspiratory and peak expiratory flow rates can be measured using a Wright peak flow meter. TLF, FRC and RV can be measured with a helium dilution technique in a closed circuit. Information can be gained when tests are repeated during standard exercise demands. Single breath nitrogen tests give information about ventilation/perfusion (V/Q) inequalities, though regional changes in V/Q need radioactive isotopes and scanning devices. Carbon monoxide diffusion capacity gives a measure of pulmonary membrane diffusion.

Blood gas analysis is necessary for baseline measurements. Dynamic compliance can be measured using an oesophageal balloon.

Ravin (1964) describes the ability to blow out a lighted match held 7·5 cm from the widely open mouth as a basis for lung function testing, particularly of peak expiratory flow rates. The widely open mouth ensures no isolated variation in linear air flow.

Of adults with FEV$_1$ above 1·6 litres, 85 per cent blew out the match, and 85 per cent of adults with FEV$_1$ below 1·6 litres did not do so. The inability to extinguish the flame is equivalent to a maximum breathing capacity (MBC) below 40 litres per minute and a maximum mid-expiratory flow rate below 0·6 litres per second. Patients with MBC below 40 litres per minute are unable to maintain ventilation above resting levels as well as those with MBC above 40. Chronic bronchitics with MBC of less than 40 can be expected to have arterial oxygen saturations below 92 per cent and raised Pa$_{CO_2}$ is seen with breathing 100 per cent oxygen. Thus, it is reasoned that most patients who can blow out the match can be expected to respond effectively to normal demands for gas exchange.

Chronic lung diseases

These cause changes in the mechanical properties of the lungs with poorly reversible expiratory flow resistance. Such chronic airways obstruction is associated with chronic bronchitis, emphysema and asthma. Obstruction to normal ventilation may be partly reversible as in asthma and chronic bronchitis or irreversible as in emphysema. General narrowing of the bronchi may be caused by tenacious secretions, oedema, infiltration in the walls, glandular hypertrophy, smooth muscle constriction or by fibrosis. Expiratory flow resistance is increased also in cases with destruction of the lung parenchyma.

With advancing age and lung disease, elastic recoil is not usually sufficient to achieve the expiratory ventilation needed and active expiration becomes necessary. Increased intrathoracic pressure is required to achieve expiration and the increased pressure has a tendency to compress large airways; when this happens, the flow through the larger airways (normally 45 per cent of the total airway resistance) determines the maximum rate of expiratory air flow which is possible.

Another important feature of the patient with chronic respiratory disease is the marked hyper-reactivity of the bronchi, which may be a cause or an effect of the condition. There is narrowing of small airways, and this usually can be reversed to some extent with isoprenaline inhalations. Diminished rigidity of the airways and the tendency to collapse are features of chronic suppurative bronchitis.

Chronic bronchitis

The striking features of this very common condition are narrowing of the bronchi with excess mucus production from a hypertrophy of mucus-secreting and goblet cells. The increased production of mucus gives a productive cough at some time of day for at least three months of two successive years. The UK has the highest mortality in the world from this condition (15 times that of Scandinavia and the USA). Cigarette smoking is the single most important factor involved in its production and the influences of smoke pollution start in childhood. The incidence increases with age, with atmospheric pollution and with lower socio-economic status. Chronic irritation and overgrowth of mucus glands, the presence of fewer cilia and irregularities of the bronchial wall mean that the mechanisms to protect the lungs are less effective. Secretions are retained and chronic infection causes fibrosis.

Simple chronic bronchitis may develop into recurrent mucopurulent bronchitis or into chronic obstructive bronchitis with air flow obstruction. When chronic bronchitis is treated with long-term antibiotics (e.g. 2 g tetracycline daily) there is no reduction in the frequency of acute exacerbations, but the duration of each is shortened.

Emphysema is a pathological, not clinical, term and is thus diagnosed either by x-ray or at post-mortem or by the characteristic pattern of clinical changes which imply underlying lung tissue destruction. The World Health Organization symposium on chronic cor pulmonale in 1963 suggests that 'Emphysema is a condition of the lung characterized by an increase beyond the normal size of the air spaces distal to the terminal bronchiole with destruction of the walls.' Emphysema is the main cause of a fall in the elastic recoil of the lungs. Destructive changes vary and it has been suggested that they occur by proteolysis of lung parenchyma by enzymes released in the lung at sites of inflammation. The reduction in elastic recoil and the subsequent restriction in function are caused by the increase in size of the air spaces so that less space exists for distension of the normal parts of the lung. Typically, the patient is aged between 50 and 60, is a smoker and has suffered from chronic bronchitis for many years. He has dyspnoea on exertion and may be wheezy, but is certainly subject to bronchial irritability especially to cold air.

Chronic lung disease has been divided into the emphysematous, restrictive type, and the bronchitic, obstructive type, though most patients with such lesions have mixed conditions with increased work of breathing, increased intrapulmonary right to left shunting and increased dead space/tidal volume ratio. It is useful to consider the two types and the extremes of the functional pathology separately.

The emphysematous ('pink puffer') type is under-weight and breathless, with an over-inflated chest (liver and cardiac dullness is reduced) and is characterized by a FVC of more than 4 seconds and an increase in TLC and RV. FEV_1, FEV/FVC and maximum expiratory flow rate (MEFR) are all reduced. There is no great change in V/Q characteristics in these patients and this is reflected in the normal Pa_{CO_2} and arterial oxygen saturation. Carbon monoxide diffusion is impaired in this group.

The bronchitic type ('blue bloater') suffers from severe dyspnoea and swelling of the ankles. He is usually plethoric, well covered and cyanosed. The chest is not so over-inflated but crepitations at the bases are audible and a prolonged expiration is evidence of the obstructive nature of the condition. Early inspiratory crackles of airways obstruction are from the proximal and larger airways, whereas the late inspiratory crackles are diffuse and gravity-dependent and are from peripheral small airways, each crackle representing the abrupt opening of one airway (Nath and Capel, 1974). The Pa_{CO_2} may be raised and the arterial oxygen saturation reduced with secondary polycythaemia (thus making cyanosis more obvious). Right ventricular failure may ensue as hypoxaemia and hypercapnia lead to reactive pulmonary vasoconstriction and cor pulmonale (Hugh-Jones, 1966). Severe V/Q changes with chronic respiratory and cardiac failure occur. Loss of CO_2 sensitivity is a common feature and ventilatory drive in the patients is maintained by the stimulus of hypoxia.

FEV_1 is the single most useful respiratory function test for initial assessment. If the value is more than 1·5 litres, moderate exercise will be tolerated and some respiratory reserve is present; between 1 and 1·5 litres the patient has some shortness of breath on exercise, and below 1 litre there is breathlessness on the slightest exertion. Early disease can be detected only by a single breath nitrogen test which identifies small airways disease.

Respiratory complications of obesity (Leading article, 1974)

Obese patients do not necessarily have primary lung disease, though this often develops later with the onset of chronic obstructive bronchitis. The severity of the pulmonary disability is not necessarily proportional to the degree of overweight. Occasionally, hypoventilation is seen. Oxygen consumption and carbon dioxide production are greater in the obese, so either at rest or on exercise they have to ventilate more. The total work of breathing is increased further because the layers of fat reduce the bellows action of the thoracic cage and the diaphragm is elevated. The chest wall component is the main contribution to the increased work of breathing.

The FRC is low because the expiratory reserve volume is reduced. CV exceeds FRC, increasing right to left intrapulmonary shunting during normal tidal ventilation and this effect is worse in the supine position. In spite of hypoxaemia, most obese patients can maintain a normal level of alveolar ventilation and a normal Pa_{CO_2}.

Ten per cent of severely obese people have the 'Pickwickian syndrome' of obesity, episodic somnolence, hypoventilation and cor pulmonale. Hypoventilation may follow a decrease in carbon dioxide sensitivity or it may just mean that the ventilatory mechanics make the patient unable to meet his ventilatory demands. Some obese patients without hypoventilation respond normally or excessively to inhaled carbon dioxide. This effect is lessened after weight loss and is possibly due to a reduction in the oxygen cost of breathing.

Fitness for general anaesthesia

With chronic obstructive or restrictive lung disease, fitness for general anaesthesia depends first on surgical considerations—urgency or the effect of the surgery on the patient, and whether functioning lung tissue will be lost or gained with the surgery. Short-term effects of surgery may be expected to include a reduction in the capacity to cough (causing sputum retention), a reduction in ventilatory capacity because of pain or narcotic analgesics, pneumothorax or pleural effusions or lung changes from anaesthesia, atelectasis or pulmonary oedema from over-transfusion. Longer term effects include reduction in ventilatory capacity or even respiratory failure if functioning lung tissue is removed. Sometimes surgery may improve mechanical factors after removal of a diseased lung with gross V/Q abnormalities.

Postoperative pulmonary complications are directly linked with preoperative assessment and treatment of chronic pre-existing lung disease. Wightman (1968) defined a postoperative lung complication if there was a productive cough, a fever of 37°C or more and signs in the chest which were not present before surgery. The incidence of such complications has not changed for 30 years, though nowadays patients are rarely rejected on the grounds of age or because of chest problems. Thus perhaps the true incidence is actually lower. The total incidence is about 5 per cent although it is 21 per cent after upper abdominal operations but only 0·6 per cent after non-abdominal or surface operations (Leading article, 1968). It is possible to make general statements about the frequency of postoperative pulmonary complications

(Ahlgren, 1968). They are mostly found, and are more severe in, patients with pre-existing lung disease. This can mean acute respiratory tract infections, colds, sinusitis or acute bronchitis as well as the chronic destructive lesions. More respiratory complications are seen after upper abdominal surgical procedures. Frequency and severity increase with the duration of surgery, though no correlation is found with the type of anaesthetic used.

Complications are less severe when patients are correctly prepared for surgery. There is a higher incidence after emergency surgery, especially that which involves gastrointestinal bleeding. Smoking, advancing age and obesity all correlate with an increased incidence of complications.

Preoperative lung function testing is mandatory to determine which patients are at risk of postoperative complications or even respiratory failure and which patients will benefit from preoperative care so that optimum conditions may be achieved for the surgery and anaesthesia. Lung function is also important to the anaesthetist as it is a guide to the uptake and distribution of anaesthetic gases.

Most commonly found is intrathoracic airways obstruction which, even in advanced chronic bronchitis and emphysema, has a reversible component. The condition also has implications because of possible loss of normal respiratory control.

Estimates of mechanical reserve

FEV_1/FVC is the commonest preoperative test; FVC of more than 4 seconds is abnormal and one of 10 seconds means severe airways obstruction. More precise information will be obtained if this is repeated after bronchial dilatation.

Stein et al. (1962) use the MEFR as a measure of ability to cough well, predicting postoperative difficulties from their results. The average normal MEFR is 280 litres per minute. The kinetic energy available to move secretions is related to the square of the velocity of flow, and a reduction in the MEFR will show an inability to produce an effective cough. FEV_1/FVC of less that 81 per cent and RV/TLC of more than half the age of the patient are indications of decreased respiratory reserve. Raised Pa_{CO_2} preoperatively is associated with complications in every case.

Postoperatively a tidal volume of 5 ml/kg body weight is a minimum (or a vital capacity of more than 15 ml/kg) (Pontoppidan, Geffin and Lowenstein, 1973).

If the figures are less, then there is a danger of alveolar hypoventilation. Rigg and Jones (1978) suggest that serial estimations of the shunt fraction should be made at rest and during exercise by measuring the physiological dead space and the pulmonary venous admixture.

The theoretical hazards of impaired ventilatory capacity are widely known but the actual level to which the FEV_1 may fall before anaesthesia is definitely contraindicated has not been worked out. Diament and Palmer (1967) suggest a ratio of less than 70 per cent, indicating that the patient is at risk of developing postoperative pulmonary complications. Stein et al. (1962) report the lowest desirable figure for FEV_1 as 0·81 litres and suggest that this in itself may constitute a hazard. They point out that patients with raised Pa_{CO_2} preoperatively always develop complications.

Assessment of breathing control

An assessment of breathing control and the response to CO_2 must be made. Any reduction in the ventilatory response to CO_2 must be interpreted in the context of the patient's respiratory capabilities—the limiting factor may be airways obstruction (a normal FEV_1 would rule this out). Patients with chronic airways obstruction and a low CO_2 response are more likely to develop respiratory failure than are patients who have a high or normal response. The measurement of the Pa_{CO_2} is a measure of alveolar ventilation, though respiratory failure must be defined in terms of Pa_{O_2} because of failure of pulmonary oxygen uptake (Pa_{O_2} less than 6·7 kPa, 50 mmHg).

Patients relying on hypoxic drive who already have a raised Pa_{CO_2} must have controlled oxygen therapy (24, 28 or 35 per cent) if progressive increases in Pa_{CO_2} and respiratory failure are not to ensue.

Exercise testing is a useful way of estimating functional reserve. Standard levels of exercise are used, though function may be measured simply after the patient has climbed one flight of stairs. Measurements of the cardiac rate, ECG, ventilatory responses and respiratory frequency can be taken and, in conjunction with blood gas analysis, pulmonary gas exchange can be estimated.

Rigg and Jones (1978) use a functional classification for cardiopulmonary reserve:

(1) Normal cardiopulmonary reserve.
(2) Reduced reserve:
   FVC or FEV_1 less than 50 per cent of predicted values;
   Pa_{CO_2} normal;
   Pa_{O_2} greater than 9·3 kPa (70 mmHg). Shunt fraction less than 10 per cent.
(3) Severe reduction in cardiopulmonary reserve:
   FVC or FEV_1;
   Pa_{CO_2} normal;
   Pa_{O_2} less than 9·3 kPa (70 mmHg). Shunt fraction > 10 per cent;
   The exercise capacity below 75 per cent of normal.
(4) No cardiopulmonary reserve. Preanaesthetic cardiac and/or pulmonary failure:
   FVC or FEV_1 less than 25 per cent of predicted;
   Arterial Pa_{CO_2} more than 6·4 kPa (50 mmHg) (mixed venous > 8 kPa (60 mmHg)),
   Arterial Pa_{O_2} less than 6·7 kPa (50 mmHg);
   Shunt fraction greater than 25 per cent.

The capacity to maintain an oxygen uptake of 1500 ml per minute shows an adequate reserve, whereas if this falls below 800 ml per minute there is great impairment of reserve and the patient constitutes a great operative risk.

Lung resections leaving FEV_1 of less than 1 litre put the patient at risk of ventilatory failure.

Lockwood (1973) showed that, after cardiothoracic surgery, both respiratory and cardiac complications were more common where abnormal lung function was demonstrated preoperatively.

It is important to use the simplest test available in an attempt to isolate those patients who are at risk from ventilatory failure postoperatively so that steps can be taken to minimize the risk by very thorough preoperative treatment. Milledge and Nunn (1975), using only FEV_1 and FVC and blood gas analysis, attempt to predict those patients who will need postoperative respiratory support. They describe three groups of patients:

(1) Those with a low FEV_1 but normal Pa_{O_2} without overt arterial hypoxaemia. No patient in this group gave any anaesthetic trouble with routine peroperative and postoperative care.

(2) Those with a low FEV_1, a low Pa_{O_2} (less than 7·3 kPa (55 mmHg)) but a normal Pa_{CO_2}. This group needed postoperative oxygen therapy.

(3) Those with a greatly reduced FEV_1, overt hypoxaemia and a Pa_{CO_2} of more than 5·9 kPa (45 mmHg). The higher the preoperative level of Pa_{CO_2} the more likely is the need for postoperative ventilation.

Thus, FEV_1 below 1 litre or 50 per cent of the predicted value means that the patient must be very carefully monitored postoperatively with serial measurements of Pa_{CO_2} and Pa_{O_2}. Certainly, Pa_{CO_2} seems to be the most important parameter of preoperative respiratory assessment and where this is increased above 6·7 kPa (50 mmHg) this often indicates the need for postoperative mechanical ventilation.

Preoperative care

The principle of preoperative care of the patient with chronic lung disease is aimed toward improving the condition as much as possible in as short a time as possible. The single most important factor is the removal of bronchial irritants, the most common of which is smoking. Improvement in function in the long term is rare for the severely disabled, but the progression of the disease may be slowed. Infection must be eradicated and the organisms most often associated with exacerbation of bronchitis are *Haemophilus influenzae* and *Pneumococcus*. Bacteriological examination of the sputum should be carried out after antibiotics are started and, in the light of clinical change and bacteriological data, the antibiotic may be changed. A dose of ampicillin of up to 4 g per day is recommended as this high dose achieves penetration into mucus and, by eliminating the infection, will produce a longer remission. Co-trimoxazole (Septrin)—a combination of trimethoprim and sulphamethoxazole—is also effective (two tablets twice daily, each containing 80 mg trimethoprim and 400 mg sulphamethoxazole). Clinical response can be expected within 48 hours.

Of the airways obstruction of chronic bronchitis, a small component can be expected to be reversible and thus respond to bronchodilator drugs. Assessment of this component can be made simply with measurements of peak flow before and after bronchodilator therapy. β-Adrenergic drugs delivered by aerosol are the most effective, and orciprenaline may be taken orally (20 mg q.d.s.) with fewer side effects. Continued over-use of aerosols, however, does not benefit and may even cause deterioration in respiratory function.

Theophylline derivatives may be useful, and choline theophyllinate may be given orally in doses of 200 mg up to four times a day.

The perioperative course of steroids is recommended for patients with severe disease, especially if an allergic component may be present. These drugs should certainly reduce a bronchiolar inflammatory state and are very effective in about 10 per cent of severe bronchitics. Improvement must be assessed objectively with serial peak flow readings because the action of corticosteroids in producing euphoria will make symptoms difficult to assess.

Thorough and frequent chest physiotherapy is a very important part of the treatment, not only to remove secretions but also to familiarize patients with techniques of physiotherapy they will need in the postoperative period. Adjuncts to physiotherapy include postural drainage and humidification of the inspired gases to loosen and thin secretions. There is no evidence that the so-called 'mucolytic' drugs are effective.

Stein and Cassara (1970) showed a marked reduction in postoperative complications in a group treated with antibiotics, bronchodilators, etc., against an untreated control group.

If there is evidence of congestive cardiac failure with oedema and a history of swelling of the ankles, and if crepitations are audible at the bases of the lungs and a raised jugular venous pressure is found, the patient needs to be digitalized and a diuresis to be provoked (frusemide, from 40 mg in the morning). Oxygen therapy may be necessary even in the preoperative phase.

Anaesthesia and the respiratory cripple

Compared to possible postoperative problems and the assessment and treatment of preoperative disease, the conduct of anaesthesia itself is relatively unimportant. Many studies have shown that the postoperative complication rate is related not to any particular anaesthetic agent or the technique used, but merely to the duration of the surgery. Care should be taken to avoid those factors which are likely to depress postoperative ventilation and increase the possibility of hypoxaemia. Sedation should be the minimum to allay apprehension, and opiate analgesics avoided where possible. Spontaneous ventilation can be maintained for patients who have a normal preoperative Pa_{CO_2}, but the anaesthetist should be aware of the possibility of further increasing the $A\text{-}aDo_2$ as CV further encroaches into tidal ventilation (Thornton, 1969). Carbon dioxide sensitivity is gradually lost as anaesthesia is deepened (it is possible that high inspired oxygen concentrations might also depress the respiratory drive) and respiratory failure follows.

Utting (1965) showed that with all patients, even those with overt respiratory failure, it is possible to maintain adequate pulmonary ventilation during anaesthesia with mechanical ventilation. It is possible to hyperventilate all patients to a lower Pa_{CO_2} than preoperative levels. Inspiratory/expiratory time ratios are best set at 1 : 2·5 or 3 to allow sufficient time for expiration (Brown and Ebert, 1963). Respiration starts again postoperatively but Pa_{CO_2} rapidly rises to preoperative levels after a few minutes of spontaneous ventilation. Care must be taken to ensure that the effects of muscle relaxants have worn off. The patient should be able to lift his head on command.

Extradural or spinal blocks are recommended for lower abdominal or pelvic surgery; continuous techniques when used to control postoperative wound pain will obviate the need for respiratory depressant analgesics. The anaesthetist must be careful not to allow the blood pressure to fall too greatly or pulmonary perfusion will be affected. Too high an extradural block will paralyse the intercostals and may cause respiratory difficulties.

In cases with a raised Pa_{CO_2} preoperatively, elective postoperative mechanical ventilation may be needed and such a course should not be regarded as a failure of the anaesthetic technique but as a logical continuation of therapy.

Postoperative problems

Surgical respiratory failure can occur in patients who have normal pulmonary function preoperatively (Morton, 1973) and such factors as disturbances of acid–base state, changes in the circulating blood volume, cardiac failure, compliance changes in the lungs and changes in V/Q characteristics are all important. Upper abdominal and thoracic incisions affect lung function, though Williams and Brenowitz (1975) showed no difference in the FRC with vertical or horizontal abdominal incisions.

Arterial hypoxaemia is the most common finding in the postoperative patient. Morton et al. (1977) found unacceptably low levels (below 7 kPa (52·5 mmHg)) in 32 per cent of patients after routine abdominal surgery. In some cases the low Pa_{O_2} persisted for three days postoperatively and the characteristics of the patients with low Pa_{O_2} were: the average age was 65 years; 80 per cent were long-term heavy smokers; 30 per cent were obese; 60 per cent had a diagnosis of chronic bronchitis; and postoperative atelectasis was demonstrated radiologically in 70 per cent of the cases. These patients were noted to have preoperative Pa_{O_2} of $8·3 \pm 0·5$ kPa ($62·3 \pm 3·8$ mmHg).

An important cause of the hypoxaemia is thought to be regional underventilation, especially at the lung bases, due to airway closure when FRC is reduced as a result of the surgical procedure (Alexander et al., 1973). Factors which affect FRC particularly include upper abdominal and thoracic operations, especially in the obese or elderly, because of the progressive loss of elastic recoil in the lungs with the ageing process, chronic bronchitics with an increase in CV, and recumbency which reduces FRC by about 10 per cent. Other causes of postoperative reduction in FRC are injury to the rib cage by accidental or surgical trauma, abdominal distension and possibly an increase in central blood volume.

Morton and Ebert (1974) also suggest that blood stasis in the lungs is an important factor causing postoperative pulmonary complications. The central blood volume is increased after trauma and left atrial pressures are often raised after major surgery. Morton and Ebert have developed x-ray techniques which are designed to show changes in pulmonary water content and which have shown increases in lung water of as much as 50 per cent. Furthermore, anaesthetic agents, especially halothane and thiopentone, depress myocardial function, increase left atrial pressure and encourage fluid to pass into the lung parenchyma (excess intravenous crystalloid or colloid will also do this). The more major the surgical procedure, the greater is the tendency to retain salt and water, and there is also the possibility of an increase in pulmonary vascular permeability. Elevation of the CV is caused by disturbances of the morphology of small airways because interstitial fluid accumulates first around smaller blood vessels and bronchi. Thus, pulmonary interstitial fluid may be partly responsible for ventilation/perfusion inequalities because of premature closing of small airways when the patient is breathing at low lung volumes in the postoperative period.

Drummond and Milne (1977) have shown that Pa_{CO_2} may rise and Pa_{O_2} always falls within hours of thoracotomy. Pa_{O_2} always falls to unacceptable levels (less than 8 kPa or 40 mmHg) if the patient is allowed to breathe room air. The fall in Pa_{O_2} is related to the preoperative value—the lower the preoperative value, the greater the postoperative fall. The pattern of response to an increased inspired oxygen concentration suggests that V/Q abnormality is responsible for the hypoxaemia. Pa_{O_2} always falls much more from the preoperative values after thoracotomy than after abdominal surgery. Hypoxia can be more severe after lobectomy than after pneumonectomy because of damage and subsequent interstitial oedema in the remaining lung on the operated side. Deep breathing and coughing improve oxygen saturation temporarily. Doxapram, which increases the tidal volume, also reduces hypoxaemia. The response to oxygen is more than predicted if the hypoxaemia is caused by shunting of blood through an unventilated lung.

All the factors causing ventilation/perfusion changes postoperatively are not known, but airway closure and decreased FRC do occur. Carbon dioxide can be retained immediately after thoracotomy, and patients are more sensitive to the respiratory depressant effects of the opiate analgesia after the thoracotomy. Thirty-five per cent oxygen is needed to restore the Pa_{O_2} to levels similar to or slightly more than those measured preoperatively. Accurate control of inspired oxygen concentration is not necessary if the preoperative Pa_{CO_2} is normal.

A contribution to the postoperative hypoxia from V/Q inequalities can be expected from a fall in cardiac output (Philbin et al., 1970). When the venous admixture is constant, a decrease in cardiac output will cause a reduction in arterial oxygenation. When pulmonary perfusion is disturbed, the physiological dead space increases and its ratio with the tidal volume is larger. The same changes occur if the tidal volume is decreased, as it may be postoperatively with pain, and this is thought to be the contributory factor to the hypoxaemia rather than regional pulmonary under-perfusion (Morton et al., 1976) unless the cardiac output falls markedly.

After V/Q inequalities, the most important cause of hypoxaemia and respiratory failure in the postoperative period is a reduction in compliance.

This reduction occurs in most patients after major abdominal surgery, and the main cause of the fall in compliance is a reduction in lung volume. Because of the effect of gravity, pleural pressure is considerably higher in the dependent parts of the thorax; near residual volume pleural pressure may exceed atmospheric pressure, and then airways close. In the elderly, as elastic recoil is reduced, pleural pressures are higher at any given lung volume. When the FRC is reduced postoperatively because of age or for surgical reasons, lung compliance will be reduced. When pleural pressure becomes positive (greater than atmospheric pressure), little or no further change in lung volume can occur due to pulmonary compression (West, 1970). When airways close in this way, compliance depends on frequency and is lower at higher respiratory rates. The previously described changes in the circulating blood volume will also cause decreases in the pulmonary compliance.

Many patients with chronic bronchitis already have a low compliance (and thus an increased work of breathing) caused by inflamed and fibrosed lungs. They can be expected to have even lower compliance postoperatively, caused by the reduction in lung volume and increase in central blood volume and also by development of atelectasis. Chronic bronchitics have narrowed airways which easily become blocked by the large quantity of mucus secretion characteristic of these patients.

Most patients with pre-existing respiratory disease will present no problem provided there has been careful preoperative, anaesthetic and postoperative management. Postoperative care includes continuation of the therapy started before surgery (antibiotics and bronchodilators), with an emphasis on chest physiotherapy to encourage deep breathing and coughing. Deep slow breathing will improve alveolar ventilation and decrease the dead space/tidal volume ratio, increase FRC and reduce the tendency to hypoxaemia. Coughing and postural drainage will clear retained secretions trapped because normal mechanisms are destroyed by disease or obtunded by anaesthesia. Respiratory depressant analgesics are to be avoided unless absolutely necessary, and reliance placed on local blocks. Breathing 50 per cent nitrous oxide with 50 per cent oxygen (Entonox) has been recommended for physiotherapy postoperatively. Together with physiotherapy, the mainstay of postoperative care is oxygen. This may be needed for up to three days postoperatively and must be given in a controlled way if Pa_{CO_2} has been raised. Ventimasks which deliver 24, 28 or 38 per cent oxygen are readily available (Simpson, 1977). If there is doubt about the status of the respiratory control, serial Pa_{CO_2} measurements must be taken with each inspired oxygen concentration until a balance between Pa_{CO_2} and Pa_{O_2} is reached.

Acute respiratory failure may be precipitated by surgery*; the Pa_{CO_2} rises in spite of care. The patient with acute CO_2 retention has impairment of consciousness or coma and is thus unable to co-operate further with the physiotherapist. It is in the context of depression of the respiratory centre by sedatives or analgesics, or when the hypoxic drive to respiration is removed by the administration of oxygen at too high a concentration, that there may be a role for respiratory stimulants. Doxapram is the most effective and has

* Treatment with bleomycin may produce serious or fatal ventilation/perfusion disturbances if the patients are anaesthetized using a high F_IO_2 or if excess crystalloids are infused. Goldiner *et al.* (1978) *British Medical Journal* **1**, 1664–7.

the widest safety margin. Because of its short duration of action, it must be given as a continuous intravenous infusion. Its action is one of central stimulation with arousal, increased respiratory efforts and, usually, coughing. In acute carbon dioxide narcosis precipitated by sedation or oxygen therapy, doxapram may rouse a comatose patient and make it possible to induce him to cough and to co-operate in the clearance of secretions. Mechanical ventilation may thus be rendered unnecessary, but it must be instituted if the patient's state of consciousness or blood gas picture deteriorates in spite of treatment.

When doxapram is given as a single dose 1·5–2 mg/kg with standard postoperative morphine analgesia, a lower pulmonary complication rate following major surgery is reported (Gawley et al., 1976). The incidence of productive cough with purulent sputum is reduced and also the doxapram group has significantly higher arterial oxygen saturation on the fifth postoperative day than the control group. The brief period of hyperventilation which the doxapram produces probably causes a reduction in the microatelectasis which is a common finding after surgery.

When serious respiratory complications are anticipated because of prolonged and major surgery, patients are probably better if postoperatively they are electively mechanically ventilated, at least for 24 hours. Intermittent positive pressure ventilation (IPPV) will allow the blood gases to be normalized though an acutely raised Pa_{CO_2} should be brought down slowly; it will allow full doses of respiratory depressant analgesic to be administered and frequent physiotherapy with expansion of the chest by manual hyperinflation and expiratory vibration. Secretions are removed by suction. After 24 hours, patients should be weaned from mechanical ventilation as soon as possible (Pontoppidan et al., 1977).

References

Ahlgren, E. W. (1968). Guidelines to the management of some respiratory problems. In: Common and uncommon problems in anesthesiology. *Clinical Anaesthesia* **3**, 197. Ed. by M. T. Jenkins, Blackwell Scientific, Oxford.

Alexander, J., Spence, A., Parikh, R. and Stuart, B. (1973). The role of airway closure in post-operative hypoxaemia. *British Journal of Anaesthesia* **45**, 34.

Brown, E. S. and Elam, J. O. (1963). Ventilation of emphysematous patients during anesthesia. *Anesthesiology* **24**, 126.

Clarke, S. (1976). Respiratory function tests. *British Journal of Hospital Medicine* **15**, 137.

Cotes, J. E. (1968) *Lung Function*. Blackwell, Oxford.

Craig, D. B., Wahba, W. M., Don, H. F., Couture, J. G. and Becklake, M. R. (1971). Closing volume and its relation to gas exchange in the seated and supine positions. *Journal of Applied Physiology* **31**, 717.

Diament, M. L. and Palmer, K. N. V. (1967). Spirometry for preoperative assessment of airways resistance. *Lancet* **i**, 1251.

Don, H. F., Wahba, W. M. and Craig, D. B. (1972). Airway closure, gas trapping and the functional residual capacity during anesthesia. *Anesthesiology* **36,** 533.

Don, H. F., Wahba, M. and Cuadrado, L. (1970). The effects of anesthesia and 100 per cent oxygen on the functional residual capacity of the lungs. *Anesthesiology* **32,** 521.

Drummond, G. B. and Milne, A. C. (1977) Oxygen therapy after thoracotomy. *British Journal of Anaesthesia* **49,** 1093.

Fletcher, C. M., Hugh-Jones, P., McNicol, M. W. and Pride, N. B. (1963). The diagnosis of pulmonary emphysema in the presence of chronic bronchitis. *Quarterly Journal of Medicine* **32,** 33.

Gawley, T. H., Dundee, J. W., Gupta, P. K. and Jones, C. J. (1976). The role of doxapram in reducing pulmonary complications after major surgery. *British Medical Journal* **1,** 122.

Hatch, D. J. and Milner, A. D. (1974). The measurement of lung function in infants and children under five years of age. *International Anesthesiology Clinics* **12,** 37.

Hugh-Jones, P. (1966) Anaesthesia for the respiratory cripple. *Proceedings of the Royal Society of Medicine* **59,** 519.

Leading article (1968). The post-operative chest. *British Medical Journal* **2,** 713.

Leading article (1974). Respiratory complications of obesity. *British Medical Journal* **2,** 519.

Lockwood, P. (1973). The relationship between preoperative lung function test results and post-operative complications in carcinoma of the bronchus. *Respiration* **30,** 105.

Milledge, J. S. and Nunn, J. F. (1975). Criteria of fitness for anaesthesia in chronic obstructive lung disease. *British Medical Journal* **3,** 670.

Morton, A. P. (1973). Surgical respiratory failure. *Anaesthesia and Intensive Care* **2,** 175.

Morton, A. P. and Ebert, B. (1974). Post-operative respiratory dysfunction: an x-ray study. *Anaesthesia and Intensive Care* **2,** 175.

Morton, A. P., Mahoney, P., Hansen, P., McBride, M. and Baker, A. B. (1976). Post-operative respiratory function: a ventilation–perfusion study. *Anaesthesia and Intensive Care* **4,** 203.

Morton, A., Mahoney, P., Hansen, P., Holling, J. and Lindley, T. (1977). Post-operative arterial hypoxaemia. *Anaesthesia and Intensive Care* **5,** 161.

Nath, A. R. and Capel, C. H. (1974). Inspiratory crackles—early and late. *Thorax* **29,** 223.

Nunn, J. F. and Panday, J. (1968). Failure to demonstrate progressive fall of arterial Po_2 during anaesthesia. *Anaesthesia* **23,** 38.

Philbin, D. M., Sullivan, S. F., Bowman, F. O., Malm, J. R. and Papper, E. M. (1970). Postoperative hypoxemia: contribution of the cardiac output. *Anesthesiology* **32,** 136.

Pontoppidan, H., Geffin, B. and Lowenstein, E. (1973). *Acute Respiratory Failure in the Adult,* p. 60. Little, Brown, Boston.

Pontoppidan, H., Wilson, R. S., Rie, M. A. and Schneider, R. C. (1977). Respiratory intensive care. *Anesthesiology* **47,** 96.

Ravin, M. B. (1964). The match test as an aid to pre-operative pulmonary evaluation. *Anesthesiology* **25**, 391.

Rigg, J. R. A. and Jones, N. L. (1978). Clinical assessment of respiratory function. *British Journal of Anaesthesia* **50**, 3.

Simpson, P. (1977). Oxygen therapy. *British Journal of Clinical Equipment* **2**, 194.

Stein, M. and Cassara, E. L. (1970). Preoperative pulmonary evaluation and therapy for surgical patients. *Journal of the American Medical Association* **211**, 787.

Stein, M., Koota, G. M., Simon, M. and Frank, H. A. (1962). Pulmonary evaluation of surgical patients. *Journal of the American Medical Association* **181**, 765.

Stone, J. G., Khambatha, H. J., Donham, R. T. and Sullivan, S. F. (1975). Pulmonary shunting during anaesthesia in man. *Canadian Anaesthetists' Society Journal* **22**, 647.

Thornton, J. A. (1969). The problem of general anaesthesia in chronic respiratory disease. *Thorax* **24**, 380.

Utting, J. E. (1965). Anaesthesia for the respiratory cripple. *Acta Anaesthesiologica Scandinavica* **9**, 29.

West, J. (1970). Ventilation: perfusion relationships. In: *Scientific Foundations of Anaesthesia*, p. 187. Ed. by C. Scurr and S. Feldman. Heinemann Medical, London.

Wightman, J. A. K. (1968). A prospective study of the incidence of postoperative pulmonary complications. *British Journal of Surgery* **55**, 85.

Williams, C. D. and Brenowitz, J. B. (1975). Ventilatory patterns after vertical and transverse upper abdominal incisions. *American Journal of Surgery* **130**, 725.

World Health Organization (1963). *Symposium: Expert Committee on Chronic Cor Pulmonale*. Technical Report Series No. 213.

Bronchial asthma

Bronchial asthma is a very common, unpredictable disorder of the respiratory tract which affects all age groups and involves episodes of breathing difficulty associated with wheezing. The condition may progress to one in which there is continuous respiratory embarrassment. The clinical picture is one of wheezing and respiratory difficulties which come in attacks, and a tight unproductive cough with very tenacious sputum. Symptoms vary from a very mild cough and wheeze—occasionally indistinguishable from a common upper respiratory tract infection—to a state of severe prostration and even death.

Asthma can be described as *spasmodic* if attacks are infrequent, *continuous* when daily wheezing is present, or *intractable* if the wheezing is constant and unrelieved by bronchodilators. *Status asthmaticus* is severe and unrelieved asthma leading to respiratory failure and systemic changes.

The lumen of the bronchioles is reduced to a varying degree by oedema of the mucosa and spasm of the smooth muscle of the bronchioles. The bronchiolar walls are thickened due to muscular hypertrophy, overgrowth of the mucous glands and an infiltration with eosinophils. The presence of eosinophils in the sputum is usually confined to the allergic type of asthma, though not necessarily so. It is a condition affecting both lungs in all fields and eventually causes bilateral obstructive hyperinflation of the lungs. The degree to which mucosal changes occur, and thus a relatively less reversible bronchospasm, is important for the treatment of the condition and also for the prognosis as far as chronic lung changes are concerned.

The usual cause of bronchial asthma in childhood is an allergic reaction (the so-called extrinsic type) in which it is possible to demonstrate allergens. There is usually a strong family history of allergy, eczema, etc., to be obtained from these patients. So-called intrinsic asthma, in which no immunological process is demonstrable, usually has its age of onset in the middle part of life, though it may start in childhood. A common finding in these patients is nasal polyps. There is no family history of allergies and skin tests are negative, but there is often an association with sensitivity to aspirin. A clear-cut distinction between the two types is not always apparent, though the distinction is useful. Occasionally, asthma can start as the extrinsic allergic type in childhood and later continue in adulthood as the intrinsic type (Jones, 1976).

Asthma, like many respiratory conditions, is so common that all anaesthetists will meet many cases during their working lives. The incidence in childhood is estimated to be 25 per 1000 children; the true incidence may be higher because, if very mild, the condition may be diagnosed as an ordinary upper respiratory tract infection or, if very severe, as recurrent attacks of pneumonitis. The morbidity and mortality are considerable and rise with the age of the patient. Exposure to a wide variety of bronchial irritants causes attacks. Emotional factors, chemical and atmospheric pollutants and viral infections are common causes of reaction in hyper-reactive bronchioles.

In older patients the differential diagnosis between asthma and left ventricular failure may be difficult because nocturnal attacks between 2 and 4 a.m. are common. This may be related to the fact that the levels of circulating corticosteroids are lowest at about that time. Carcinoid syndrome is a rare cause of attacks of bronchospasm.

Half of the children with asthma can expect to be free of it by adulthood, but 5–10 per cent continue with severe disability and severe attacks can occur decades later.

The incidence of unexpected deaths from asthma is increasing throughout the world. For one series in the UK an eightfold increase in mortality was reported over the decade 1964–1974. Two-thirds of the patients were taking some sort of steroid preparation but these had been in use for at least ten years before the great rise in mortality. Epidemiological studies in Australia and Europe linked the rise with the use of bronchodilators delivered from pressurized aerosol canisters (Speizer, Doll and Heaf, 1968). In fact, 84 per cent of the patients who died were using one form or another of aerosol bronchodilator therapy (see below). Toxicity of the Freon propellant has been suggested as a cause and, though this has not been completely ruled out, it is unlikely.

Allergic asthma is the most common and most important form of spontaneous human hypersensitivity. The avoidance of the allergens where possible plays a great part in the treatment of this condition. Atopic antibodies appear after sensitization to certain environmental substances which can be either haptens (with serum proteins) or complete antigens, the commonest being pollen, house dust, house-dust mites, insect stings and drugs such as aspirin and penicillin. The capacity to produce large amounts of IgE is one of the main features of the atopy syndrome. IgE can be measured and is found attached to the basophils and the mast cells, though in up to 20 per cent of patients IgG is the causal factor. It is possible to conduct skin and mucous membrane tests for specific sensitization in allergic patients to identify and therefore to be able to avoid the allergens to which they have become sensitized.

The pathological features of asthma are caused by allergic mechanisms which are as yet not fully understood. The interaction between antigen and antibody on the surface of the mast cell is followed by the release of certain active chemical mediators—histamine, slow-reacting substance A (SRS-A) and eosinophil chemotactic factor of anaphylaxis (ECF-A). The action of the released substances on the receptor cells causes contraction of the bronchiolar smooth muscle cells and the relaxation and increased permeability of cells lining the small pulmonary blood vessels. Mast cells, the main site of release of the chemical mediators following antibody–antigen reaction, contain dense granules within the cytoplasm but which are attached to the cell surface with microtubules. The granules contain stored histamine, and 5-HT–SRS-A is not stored in the granules but is generated in response to certain stimuli. The number of mast cells is reduced in asthmatics and those that are found contain fewer granules. It has been shown that degranulation is most likely to occur in the allergic subject.

The mast cells are found mainly in the submucosa but also in the bronchiolar lumen; it is thought that antibody–antigen reaction takes place in the lumen of the bronchiole and the chemical mediators are subsequently reabsorbed.

IgE is a heat-labile antibody which is fixed to tissue cells and is also free in small quantities. It is the antibody on the cells which renders them sensitive to antigen.

Antibody–antigen reaction allows Ca^{2+} to enter the cell and this in turn causes contraction of the cellular microfilaments, leading to extrusion of the granules and their contents from the microtubules. Other factors which may be operative to influence granule release are:

(1) Activation of the enzyme serine-esterase after antibody–antigen reaction.

(2) Release of granules also depends on an intact glycolytic pathway.

(3) Mediator release is slowed by the presence of cyclic AMP.

(4) Disodium cromoglycate inhibits granular release by some unknown mechanism (Orange and Austen, 1973).

Histamine

Histamine is stored in mast cells. It is rapidly released after the antibody–antigen reaction and acts to contract smooth muscle in bronchial arteries and veins and to increase capillary permeability. Asthmatics appear to be more sensitive to the effects of histamine, and it is possible that this is part of the syndrome of atopy. Histamine seems to have both direct and indirect action and the latter is mediated by both a vagal reflex because this may be partly blocked by atropine and an α-adrenergic reflex because α-adrenergic blockers (e.g. phentolamine) partly block the constrictor response. Antihistamine drugs also block the response.

SRS-A and ECF-A

SRS-A is an unsaturated, low molecular weight hydroxy acid which is not blocked by antihistamines. ECF-A is a peptide isolated from human lung which has been sensitized to IgE and then challenged with a specific antigen.

Intracellular cyclic AMP

A further substance which may play a part in the bronchiolar constriction is intracellular cyclic AMP. An increase in this organic phosphate causes relaxation of bronchial smooth muscle. At any time, the cellular concentration of cyclic AMP depends on a balance between its production and its destruction, both of which are subject to various factors which may operate from time to time. β-Sympathetic activity causes activation of the enzyme, adenyl cyclase, which governs the production of cyclic AMP, and there exists a reverse relationship between cyclic AMP and histamine (and SRS-A).

Constant autopsy findings with bronchial asthma are extreme over-inflation of the lungs, with emphysematous blebs which increase in size with age. The lungs feel stiff and rubbery. Varying degrees of atelectasis are present and a striking finding is the presence of tenacious mucous plugs in the bronchioles, with or without infection. Microscopic findings are in increased thickness and hyalinization of the basement membrane and hypertrophy of mucous and goblet cells of bronchial and bronchiolar mucosa, causing the typical 'plugs'. Bronchiolectasis of the respiratory bronchioles can lead to panlobar emphysema with airways obstruction, but without any alveolar obstruction. There is patchy loss of the cilia and thus mechanisms for clearing secretions are less efficient and the mucosa may become redundant, almost polypoid in appearance. Peribronchiolar oedema adds to the reduction in the luminar diameter. Structural changes in the smooth muscle are difficult to detect—so much so that some investigators have actually questioned whether muscle spasm is actually a feature of asthma, though how the reversible element is relieved, especially with the use of bronchodilators, could not be explained.

In older people the lungs are more fibrous, with thinning of alveoli, emphysema and rupture of alveoli. The most severely affected asthmatics have usually been treated with steroids, so many of the pathological changes may be attributable to prolonged steroid therapy.

Lung function tests in bronchial asthmatics show impairment of function but this may fluctuate widely. Narrowing of the small airways means that they will close on expiration at a greater lung volume than normal. Thus, FRC and RV are larger in asthmatics even between attacks . If the physiological dead space volume increases as it tends to do, progressively, alveolar ventilation must be maintained by increases in tidal volume or frequency of ventilation.

Palmer and Kelman (1975) describe a group of 35 patients (average age 28 years) whose average ratio FEV_1 to FVC was 81 per cent, which is within the normal range for the age group. Even with this ratio within the normal range, the patients were found to have arterial hypoxaemia and hypocapnia, secondary to lung hyperinflation—and pulmonary abnormalities of bronchial asthma are not always detectable by simple spirometric tests. However, FEV_1/FVC above 70 per cent is usually taken to exclude significant airways obstruction or other pulmonary dysfunction in bronchial asthma. The evidence for lung hyperinflation is an increase in RV/TLC to 113 per cent and RV to 118 per cent of predicted values. Increases in FRC are usually seen as compensation for increased airways resistance (Weng and Levison, 1969).

The maximum ventilatory volume (MVV) is limited by flow during expiration, just as is FEV_1, and the two correlate ($FEV_1 \times 30$ is approximately equal to MVV). Lung compliance—a measure of the elastic recoil and surface tension properties of the lungs—is often normal in asthma until there are emphysematous changes, when compliance may be decreased. Compliance is decreased if pulmonary fibrotic changes are present. Lung units not taking part in ventilation cause a reduction in compliance proportional to the decrease in vital capacity. Airways resistance, which is the pressure difference between the alveoli and the mouth per unit of gas flow, is very important because of its relation to the work of breathing. There is an inverse relationship between the airways resistance and the volume of the lung at which it is measured. Normally the resistance is diminished with lung inflation because the airway diameter increases, and, conversely, as the lung inflation is reduced towards the RV of the lung at which airways close off, there is a marked increase in airways resistance. In the case of the asthmatic, the narrower airways tend to close at a volume equal to or more than the FRC, and this changes the relation between resistance of the airways and the lung volume. The asthmatic breathes at a higher respiratory level to minimize airways resistance (Fig. 2.2).

The work of breathing, which at its most simple is a product of the pressure change and the lung volume change, is usually increased in the asthmatic because the resting level of respiration is increased. Thus for the same inspired volume more work must be done against elastic recoil because the lungs are less compliant when more distended. Work is also increased with an increase in airways resistance.

The main increase in resistance of the airway in asthmatics is at the level of the small airways (< 2 mm diameter) and these constitute 10 per cent of the resistance in the normal subject. Forty-five per cent of the resistance is contributed by the larger airways (45 per cent by the extrathoracic, upper airways) which are important functionally because they collapse with extra-pulmonary pressure and may thus be able to control expiratory flow or be the limiting factor for expiratory flow in certain disease states (e.g. emphy-sema).

Small airways disease can be detected using single breath nitrogen tests

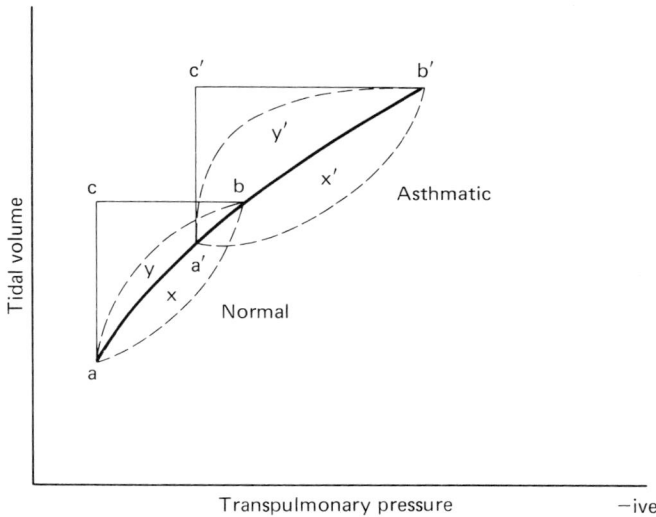

Fig. 2.2   Volume/pressure curve of the normal and the asthmatic patient. a, a', b, b' is curved implying a decrease in compliance with increase in lung volume.
Work during inspiration against elastic recoil is represented by area a b c and that done against airway resistance, X.
The asthmatic lung is more inflated and work on inspiration is represented by a', b', c'+x'. Work during expiration is represented by y and y' in the normal and asthmatic respectively.

or by other tests which demonstrate ventilation/perfusion (V/Q) inequalities (e.g. helium distribution).

Because asthma occurs in attacks, though pulmonary function is not neces-sarily normal between them, respiratory function testing usually involves tests of bronchiolar lability; the degree to which this is present is important for it enables the physician to treat the patient most effectively. Exercise test-ing with measurement of FEV_1 is the most reliable way of demonstrating bronchiolar lability. If the FEV_1 is normal at rest but there is a strong history of attacks, minimal mucosal changes will be present. Exercise causes initial bronchiolar dilatation, possibly by release of catecholamines, followed by con-striction, the mechanism for which is not known but may involve acidosis and release of constricting substances. In the asthmatic, β-adrenergic blockade causes bronchiolar constriction at rest (a contraindication to the use of these agents) and it appears therefore that these patients depend on β activity for maintenance of relaxation of airways (McNeill and Ingram, 1966). The bronchiolar cell is subject to influences causing both constriction and dilatation and this balance is upset during exercise. The FEV_1 is reduced during an exercise-induced attack but will return to near normal after treatment with a bronchodilator agent.

The proportion of smooth muscle in the bronchiolar wall is large in relation to the total wall thickness and is supplied by sympathetic and parasympathetic supply. An increase in parasympathetic tone causes bronchoconstriction in asthmatics, and atropine will reduce the airways resistance.

Direct influences include hypoxia, which causes constriction of bronchioles and pulmonary arterioles, thus tending to restore inequalities of ventilation/perfusion. Carbon dioxide has little or no direct effect.

Drugs used in asthma

Bronchodilators

Bronchodilators are of the xanthine or sympathomimetic amine groups of drugs.

Adrenergic activity is divided into α activity, which is a vasoconstrictor action, and β activity, which consists of positive inotropic and chronotropic effects on the heart ($\beta1$) and bronchodilatation ($\beta2$).

Adrenaline (has both α- and β-adrenergic effects) is occasionally used for a severe asthmatic attack by subcutaneous injection of 0·1–0·3 ml of 1 in 1000 adrenaline at 30-minute intervals until there is relief of symptoms. Relaxation of bronchioles occurs in 5–10 minutes and lasts from 30 to 60 minutes. Serious cardiovascular side effects may occur, including dangerous arrhythmias especially in the presence of hypoxia (Palmer and Diament, 1967).

Isoprenaline has both $\beta1$ and $\beta2$ activity and is active when instilled into the airway in doses of 0·5 ml of 0·5–1·0 per cent solution. Relaxation can be expected in 1–2 minutes and will last for 10–30 minutes.

Salbutamol

Salbutamol (Ventolin) is a β-adrenergic stimulant drug available as a pressurized aerosol. Structurally, it is an analogue of isoprenaline with a substitution of a 3-hydroxy group and because of this is not inactivated by catechol-O-methyltransferase and is active via the oral route (unlike isoprenaline). A large proportion of inhaled drug is swallowed and partially inactivated in the gastrointestinal tract. The cardiac chronotropic effects of salbutamol are ten times less than those of isoprenaline but is equipotent as a bronchodilator in man. The proportions of $\beta1$ to $\beta2$ activity differ with the experimental animal used for testing. In man, cardiac stimulation does not occur at doses which produce effective bronchodilatation. Salbutamol is only a partial agonist on cardiac muscle, and this differs from isoprenaline and orciprenaline which are both full agonists.

If administered orally, the peak level lasts for 3–5 hours. The FEV_1 is at a maximum within 15 minutes of inhalation, but returns to the baseline in about 4 hours. Salbutamol 100 μg and isoprenaline 100 μg each can increase the FEV_1 by 30 per cent, which can maintain effective bronchodilatation for 1 hour in the case of isoprenaline but for 3 hours with salbutamol. This effect is probably related to the gastrointestinal absorption and effective activity of the latter drug.

The most troublesome side effect of salbutamol is a tremor seen in 20 per cent of patients, the incidence of which depends on the dosage and is more frequent when administered orally.

Salbutamol is prepared in tablet form (2–4 mg) or syrup for children (2 mg in 5 ml), a suitable dose being 1–2 mg for a child under 6 years of age The Ventolin aerosol contains 200 inhalations each of 100 μg, the dose of which is one to two puffs 4-hourly but not more than eight in a 24-hour period.

Orciprenaline

Orciprenaline is not a catechol, so is effective when taken by mouth. Like salbutamol, it has mostly $\beta2$ effects and gives effective bronchodilatation for up to 3 hours. The dose is up to 20 mg four times per day, or aerosol administration of 750 μg no more than eight times each 24-hour period. On comparing the recommended therapeutic dose of two puffs of either salbutamol or orciprenaline, salbutamol produces a larger increase in FEV_1 than orciprenaline.

The striking increase in the mortality from acute asthmatic attacks during the 1960s has been mentioned earlier in this chapter. The increase coincided with the use of aerosols.

Isoprenaline

Isoprenaline, which relaxes smooth muscle, increases cardiac output and dilates pulmonary vasculature, causes an increase in minute ventilation and dead space/tidal volume ratio, thus intensifying V/Q inequalities. This is a possible explanation of the falls in Pa_{O_2} of up to 2 kPa (15 mmHg) seen with the use of isoprenaline even in the face of symptomatic relief of bronchospasm. It is not possible to correlate changes in Pa_{O_2} with changes in FEV_1. In a patient who already has a low Pa_{O_2} during an attack of asthma, a further fall may be disastrous; arrhythmias induced by the $\beta1$ action of isoprenaline on the heart and in the presence of hypoxia may be the cause of death in some of these patients. Poynter and Spurling (1971) have shown that hearts working against an increased load are particularly susceptible to the effects of β stimulation.

The isoprenaline effect causing a fall in Pa_{O_2} in spite of symptomatic relief of symptoms can be explained in terms of further disorder of V/Q in the lungs. However, the same falls in Pa_{O_2} seen with salbutamol are not so easy to explain; they are smaller and less consistent than with isoprenaline and may be a reflection of the weaker $\beta 1$ cardiac effects of the former. The mixture of phenylephrine and isoprenaline in the Medihaler duo does not have the effect of reducing the Pa_{O_2} or increasing Pa_{CO_2} (Alliott *et al.*, 1972). The phenylephrine acts on α receptors and may protect against the non-selective pulmonary vasodilatation and against the increase in cardiac output which occurs with $\beta 2$ stimulators. It also aids bronchodilatation by delaying isoprenaline absorption. Beta blockade can prevent isoprenaline-induced increase in hypoxaemia.

Another suggestion to explain the increase in mortality is that isoprenaline in its metabolism is partly converted to 3-methoxyisoprenaline which is a weak β antagonist and this may contribute to cardiac arrhythmias, the effect of which will be intensified in the presence of hypoxia. Overdosage with sympathomimetic amines causes failure to relax smooth muscle and often increased constriction which is also explicable on the basis of an increase in this metabolite. Great clinical improvement is seen when aerosols are withdrawn from this group of patients who have been greatly over-using them and in whom bronchodilatation has been unrelieved.

Aminophylline

Aminophylline inhibits phosphodiesterase which converts cyclic 3,5-AMP to 5-AMP thereby increasing the action of sympathomimetic amines (hence the combined pharmaceutical preparation with ephedrine). Given intravenously, it increases the rate and depth of respiration, causes relaxation of bronchiolar smooth muscle, an increase in myocardial contractility, a fall in venous pressure and an increase in cardiac output. The FEV_1 increases at once and effective bronchodilatation is sustained over an 8-hour period. The effect on gas transfer is variable (like that of the sympathomimetic amines); it may relieve bronchoconstriction but can increase or decrease Pa_{O_2} (Rees *et al.*, 1967). Treatment with aminophylline needs monitoring to see the most effective way of administration and necessary frequency. Aminophylline is usually given by intravenous injection of 250 to 500 mg over 5 minutes. Fast injection can cause profound hypotension, and sudden death has been reported. Suppositories are available, but the only non-irritant oral preparation is choline theophyllinate in doses of 100 to 400 mg, 4 times a day.

Disodium cromoglycate

Disodium cromoglycate (Intal) specifically inhibits allergic reactions in the respiratory tract and is used with great effect in patients with hay fever and with bronchial asthma of the extrinsic type. Disodium cromoglycate is an inert substance of which about 10 per cent of an inhaled dose is absorbed from the lungs and is excreted unchanged. It is free from side effects and has no direct bronchodilatory or anti-inflammatory activity. Its primary site of action is on the mast cell to stabilize it and to prevent the release of the mediator-containing granules. It does not prevent the weal and flare reaction in the skin. Doses of 20 mg (Spincaps) are delivered from a special inhaler (Spinhaler); as it is an expensive drug, it should be used with discrimination.

The standard initial dose of 80 mg per day can often be reduced to 40 mg without precipitating a recurrence of asthma. The effective action of the drug (and the minimum level of dosage) can be shown by its inhibiting effect on bronchoconstriction following inhalation of an allergen (provocation test). Fifty per cent of children benefit from disodium cromoglycate, especially those whose asthma is labile, though it is unsuitable if attacks occur at intervals of more than one month. The drug should not, however, be denied to a patient with asthma classed as intrinsic, because 1 in 3 of these patients also benefit. An improvement will be seen within four weeks of treatment. As mucosal disease and mucous plugging increase, there is less indication for the use of disodium cromoglycate.

Asthma induced by exercise or voluntary hyperventilation can be inhibited by sodium cromoglycate, and a good long-term response to this drug can be predicted if a reduction in FEV_1 is recorded after 2 minutes of hyperventilation. Patients with clumps of eosinophils in the sputum also seem to respond to the drug.

Disodium cromoglycate is unsuitable for treatment of attacks; when these occur, it should be withdrawn and salbutamol substituted.

Parasympatholytic drugs

Though there is limited knowledge of the sensory receptors in the airways, it is known that bronchial motor innervation is cholinergic and the sympathetic system supplies only the vascular smooth muscle. Atropine, which blocks the muscarinic action of acetylcholine at the cholinergic nerve endings, produces bronchiolar muscle cell relaxation and inhibition of mucosal secretions. Reflex bronchoconstriction in response to non-antigenic irritant stimuli is prevented by parasympathetic block. Atropine partly blocks antigen-induced bronchospasm. Histamine bronchospasm is partly inhibited by atropine because some of its release is mediated via a vagal reflex, but the relative ineffectiveness in an asthmatic attack and in the prevention of bronchoconstriction induced by exercise must mean that other receptors are involved.

Sch 1000

Sch 1000 or ipratropium bromide (Atrovent) is a new tropane alkaloid derivative which has been shown to be very efficient in suppressing or reducing bronchoconstriction initiated by vagal reflexes due to airways irritation, cigarette smoking, etc. Suppression of constriction with exposure to allergens is not so clear-cut, but is better in children than in adults (Engelhardt and Klupp, 1975).

Atropine-like drugs have been previously neglected because of the fear of reducing the quantity and increasing the viscosity of sputum and thus worsening the situation with tenacious secretions. However, in clinical doses there are no adverse effects on the mucociliary function. No important haemodynamic or cardiac effects are seen, nor is there any deleterious effect on the V/Q ratio because of side effects on the pulmonary vascular bed.

Thus those who gain the most benefit from the use of Sch 1000 (ipratropium bromide) are the non-allergic bronchitics. In this group, any suppression of mucus without increasing its viscosity might also be desirable.

Inhalation is the most suitable method of administration, as the most effective concentration is delivered locally to the smooth muscle of the bronchial tree without producing anticholinergic side effects after absorption into the blood stream.

Steroid therapy

Steroids modify the course of hypersensitivity reactions, lessening their effect and reducing inflammation. The mechanism is not known but there seems to be little or no action on the formation of antibody and no direct action on antigen. Histamine formation is inhibited and blood histamine levels are reduced. Steroids may have a direct effect on smooth muscle, but they definitely reduce inflammatory reactions of the bronchioles, reduce oedema, mucus secretion and bronchial reactivity.

When asthma cannot effectively be controlled by disodium cromoglycate or relieved by a sympathomimetic bronchodilator, the most effective treatment is a corticosteroid.

ACTH, which causes the release of hydrocortisone and corticosterone from the adrenal cortex, is given by intramuscular injection of a depot preparation (e.g. with zinc) to give a prolonged action so that no more than two or three weekly injections are necessary. The response to treatment with reversal of mucosal abnormalities is variable, occasionally being better or even worse than with hydrocortisone. The main advantage of its use in children is that growth retardation is less, and also the adrenal cortex remains active (Friedman and Strang, 1966). Side effects include those seen with glucocorticoids—osteoporosis—etc., but more serious allergic reactions from the corticotrophic hormone have been described. Antibody formation may inactivate ACTH.

The primary use of corticosteroids is for the treatment of the acute attack with a short course beginning with hydrocortisone, 1–200 mg by intravenous injection. After 40 mg prednisolone orally, the first detectable effect on the PEFR and FEV_1 is seen within 3 hours and the maximum effect at about 9 hours; 200 mg hydrocortisone intravenously has an effect in 1 hour with a peak at 5 hours. Barbiturates and phenytoin accelerate the metabolism of cortisol and may increase asthmatic symptoms.

Failure of growth in children is a risk with maintenance therapy though stunting of growth is a feature of severe asthma anyway. Alternate day therapy may be possible, though Jones (1976) suggests that the risk of growth failure is small if daily prednisolone dosage does not exceed 3 mg/m^2 of body surface area. The other side effects of the steroids are well known and include mental disturbances in children, negative nitrogen balance, diabetes and hypoglycaemia.

Once an asthmatic has been put on a course of steroids, every attempt to withdraw it may cause a recurrence of asthma. Many attempts have been made to find a corticosteroid which would be active when inhaled but would not have side effects. None was successful until betamethasone, a steroid with topical activity, was tried. Betamethasone valerate in doses of 100 μg per puff or its chlorinated analogue beclomethasone dipropionate, 50 μg per puff, are delivered from an aerosol. A large proportion of the dose is swallowed and absorbed from the gut. It effectively suppresses asthma without deleterious side effects. Aerosol steroid without systemic side effects could be substituted in patients on maintenance prednisolone of 10 mg per day or less. If the dose of beclomethasone is increased above 1000 μg per day it is absorbed sufficiently to cause suppression of the hypothalamic adrenal cortex axis and thus higher doses of the aerosol would have no advantage over corticosteroids given orally.

Regular intake is essential because it is a preventative drug. In 10 per cent of patients the occurrence of oral thrush necessitates the drug being withdrawn, temporarily at least. Care must be taken when patients are changing from prolonged courses of oral steroids to topical ones, as depression of the adrenal cortex may be present. Such patients should be given oral prednisolone if they are unable (e.g. with acute respiratory infection) to take the topical steroid by inhalation.

Antihistamines

Synthetic competitive antihistamine compounds such as mepyramine or promethazine specifically prevent free histamine from affecting cells by blocking the receptors upon which histamine normally exerts its effect. However, bronchial asthma is rarely modified by antihistamines, as histamine is only a minor factor in causing the bronchoconstriction in this condition.

Analgesics and asthma (Leading article, 1973)

Asthmatics who are sensitive to aspirin usually have developed the asthma after the age of 30 and may also suffer from nasal polyps. Aspirin sensitivity giving urticaria in which aspirin is a hapten may not be the same mechanism as with asthma. For the aspirin-sensitive asthmatic no analgesic can unequivocally be regarded as safe because sensitivity is often seen also with indomethacin, paracetamol and pentazocine. Because of the difference in molecular structure, cross-reactivity between these various compounds is rather unlikely. An interaction between the analgesics and prostaglandins in the lung has been suggested. Prostaglandin F is a bronchoconstrictor substance and E is a bronchodilator. The balance between the two may be disturbed in the asthmatic so that the subject is abnormally sensitive to agents which affect one or other prostaglandin.

If wheezing develops, isoprenaline and aminophylline will be needed; for patients in whom analgesia is necessary (e.g. arthritis), a trial in hospital may be necessary to discover which analgesics may be safely administered.

Oxygen therapy

Asthmatic patients suffer from varying degrees of hypoxaemia even between attacks. It has been shown that this can be aggravated by sympathomimetic bronchodilators even in the face of symptomatic relief. The main cause of arterial hypoxaemia is an increase in right to left intrapulmonary shunting because of regional hypoventilation. Differing small airways resistance worsens as the respiratory rate increases. Airway closure adds to the venous admixture when FRC decreases with anaesthesia or sedation. The work of breathing can take up to half the total body oxygen consumption. Further hypoxaemia will be caused by increasing V/Q inequalities if the cardiac output is reduced as it will be secondary to hypoxia, hypovolaemia or acidosis.

In an asthmatic attack the Pa_{O_2} falls proportionally with the degree of airways obstruction and increases in lung hyperinflation as shown by falls in FEV_1 and the ratio of RV/TLC (Leading article, 1976). In spite of falls in Pa_{O_2}, the minute ventilation and alveolar ventilation are increased, causing a lower Pa_{CO_2} and a mild respiratory alkalosis. The Pa_{CO_2} is set low by both hypoxaemia and increased stimulation from lung receptors. As the condition worsens and smaller airways become completely occluded by oedema, spasm and retained tenacious secretions, alveolar ventilation falls in spite of increasing respiratory frequency. Pa_{CO_2} rises to normal and will rise further if deterioration continues. This state is always associated with falling Pa_{O_2}, with the patient breathing air sometimes to very low levels. The effect of the oxygen dissociation curve is important at this stage. When the Pa_{CO_2} is low, the curve is shifted to the left, and severe hypoxaemia can be present without clinical evidence of cyanosis; the clinical guide is a pulse rate of more than 130 per minute, and the inability of the patient to speak because of 'breathlessness'. These patients are already functioning in the steep part of the curve so that a small further fall in Pa_{O_2} will result in a much greater fall in oxygen saturation.

It is well known that, in patients with chronic bronchitis and chronic hypercapnia where the central drive to ventilation is depressed, the hypoxaemic drive is necessary to maintain alveolar ventilation. Controlled oxygen therapy must be administered to these patients to strike a balance between correcting the hypoxia and not obtunding the respiratory drive. It is often thought that asthmatics are hypoxaemic without hypercapnia and the respiratory control is normal so that oxygen can be freely given without risking depression of ventilatory drive. If there is any doubt, the patient's response to controlled oxygen therapy must be assessed by serial measurements of Pa_{CO_2}. In practice, hypoxic and hypercapnic ventilatory drives may be reduced in asthmatics and the effect is worsened as airways obstruction worsens. Both adults and children with severe asthma may have respiratory acidosis, which will be made more severe by indiscriminate use of oxygen. This may be because the ventilatory response to carbon dioxide is reduced when the mechanical work of breathing is greatly increased, though the range of response to carbon dioxide is wide in normal people as well as in asthmatics. It might be that the patients whose Pa_{CO_2} increases are those with blunted responses to carbon dioxide even when well. If an asthmatic patient needs oxygen, it is wise to give controlled oxygen at the outset—24, 28 and then 35 per cent—with constant monitoring of the clinical effect and with frequent blood gas measurements.

Many patients die in an acute attack of asthma because eventually they become too exhausted to maintain alveolar ventilation, and it is often necessary to institute mechanical ventilation to treat patients with status asthmaticus. Such active intervention is required if there is deterioration of the clinical state despite adequate medical treatment—which would include steroids (usually hydrocortisone 4 mg/kg 2-hourly intravenously) and salbutamol 3·6 μg/kg per minute intravenously (with monitoring of blood pressure as this may rise). A rising Pa_{CO_2} even with the use of controlled oxygen therapy is usually also a sign of failing respiratory reserve. The third important indication for mechanical ventilation is cyanosis in spite of oxygen therapy (Pa_{O_2} below 8 kPa (60 mmHg) in spite of high Fi_{O_2}). By this stage little wheezing can be heard because so little air is being shifted. A chest x-ray, to rule out pneumothorax before intubation and mechanical ventilation is instituted, is important though this will only affect the decision to insert a chest drain as well as an endotracheal tube.

The patient is intubated after sedation with diazepam and relaxation with suxamethonium 1 mg/kg. Nasotracheal intubation is used for children. An asthmatic with hypercarbia and a great drive to ventilation will need muscular paralysis, possibly with the use of pancuronium if he is to be mechanically ventilated in an optimal way. The volume-cycled flow-generating type of ventilator is preferable because of the very high ventilatory pressures needed to achieve an adequate tidal volume. A slow respiratory rate with a slow inspiratory time are necessary to achieve optimal distribution of gas. A prolonged expiratory time is also necessary and can be judged by auscultation of the chest so that inspiration does not begin until expiration is at an end, or air trapping with over-inflation of the lungs will ensue.

Although the tidal volume may be adequate, the minute ventilation may not be because of the prolonged expiratory phase which is necessary. The initial blood gas determinations may well show the Pa_{CO_2} not to be reduced towards normal. The inspired gases must be fully humidified and, in addition, normal saline is instilled down the endotracheal tube before suctioning to remove tenacious secretions. Medical treatment with steroids, bronchodilatation (intravenously and/or via the endotracheal tube) and antibiotics should continue. Serial blood gas analysis will be a guide to management of the ventilator and will show when improvements occur. When the bronchiolar muscle relaxes, trapped bronchiolar secretions are released which must be very frequently suctioned. Pneumothorax is a common complication and must be borne in mind during intermittent positive pressure ventilation (IPPV).

Controlled ventilation is continued until bronchospasm is relieved, medical treatment is reduced, and blood gases and respiratory parameters are normal.

Anaesthesia and asthma

The anaesthetist presented with an asthmatic patient of any age must know from the history—the type of asthma, the severity of attacks, how often they occur and what provokes them—whether there is a previous anaesthetic history, whether there are known drug allergies and what medication is currently being used to control the asthma. Simple respiratory function testing should be performed and FEV_1 and MEFR are the most useful, and blood gas analysis might be of value as a baseline investigation.

With abnormal results or if the patient has severe asthma, the possibility of delaying the surgery should be sought in order that adequate preoperative preparations can be made. There is evidence that there is a decrease in the incidence of per- and postoperative complications in asthmatics treated preoperatively with physiotherapy, bronchodilatation and antibiotics if infection is present (Prinkman and Whitcomb, 1959). The use of steroids should also be considered for patients with moderate to severe pulmonary insufficiency: 10–25 mg q.d.s. of oral prednisone for 4 days preoperatively and 100 mg during the operation. The dose may then be tailed off. Schnider and Papper (1961) suggest that effective preoperative preparation makes wheezing patients as safe for anaesthesia and surgery as asymptomatic cases not on treatment.

Premedication should logically consist of atropine with a sedative agent and perhaps an antihistamine agent as well. Aminophylline suppositories may be given at this stage.

There exists a 6–7 per cent incidence of bronchospasm during anaesthesia in patients with a history of asthma. Regional anaesthesia does not cause a reduced incidence nor does it protect against the development of postoperative complications.

The dangers of bronchospasm include hypoxia and hypercapnia, which cause pulmonary oedema even with a normal myocardium and severe decompensation in a patient with a poor myocardium. The risk of pneumothorax and postoperative atelectasis is increased.

The effect of the maintenance anaesthetic agent is important. Diethyl ether has traditionally been used to end attacks of bronchospasm during anaesthesia and this agent, when used in large quantities, will improve 60 per cent of patients with bronchospasm. Halothane relaxes bronchial musculature; clinical experience shows that this agent improves asthma and is therefore the agent of choice for establishment of general anaesthesia (perhaps before endotracheal intubation), and for treating an attack of bronchospasm should it occur (Gold and Helrich, 1962). Anaesthesia of moderate depth will also obtund reflexes from the periphery involved in surgical stimulation which might cause bronchospasm; for example, manipulation of the lung hilum, of the vagina or of the rectum (Smith and Volpitto, 1960).

If bronchospasm does occur, then the level of anaesthesia should be deepened with halothane, and aminophylline 250 mg by slow intravenous injection should be given. Ventilation with 100 per cent oxygen may be necessary. Isoprenaline 0·5 ml of 0·5 per cent solution may be instilled down the endotracheal tube.

Spontaneous breathing techniques should probably be used only for short cases. The mechanism by which airway closure occurs during anaesthesia even in the 'normal' patient is exaggerated in the asthmatic. Mechanical ventilation should ensure that the raised resting level of the asthmatic is maintained or airway closure will encroach further into normal tidal breathing, with increased right to left intrapulmonary shunting and the possibility of severe hypoxaemia. A mechanical ventilator should be set at an inspiratory/expiratory time ratio (where this is possible) of 1 : 2·5 or 3 to allow time for full expiration. The ganglion-blocking agent, trimetaphan (Arfonad), may cause the release of histamine and would be contraindicated for the production of induced hypotension in an asthmatic; sodium nitroprusside is an alternative drug. Care must be taken with the use of anticholinesterase drugs at the end of the operation, and adequate doses of atropine must precede the injection of prostigmine.

Ketamine hydrochloride has been shown to increase lung compliance and lower airways resistance in patients with bronchospasm (Corssen et al., 1972). The mechanism of action is not fully understood, but its effect is dose-related and may be due to catecholamine release. Ketamine has been used to terminate attacks of bronchospasm during anaesthesia and also to treat severe cases of status asthmaticus in which conventional medical treatment has failed (Fisher, 1977).

Anaesthetic care for the asthmatic should be directed toward prevention of attacks rather than treatment when they have occurred. Drying of the secretions and vagal blockage are necessary, as is adequate anaesthesia at all times. Care must be taken with drugs which have been implicated in causing histamine-related bronchospasm.

References

Alliott, R. J., Lang, B. D., Rawson, D. R. W. and Leckie, W. J. H. (1972). Effects of salbutamol and isoprenaline/phenylephrine in reversible airways obstruction. *British Medical Journal* 1, 539.

Corssen, G., Cutierrez, J., Reves, J. A. and Huber, F. C. (1972). Ketamine in the anesthetic management of asthmatic patients. *Anesthesia and Analgesia: Current Researches* 81, 588.

Engelhardt, A. and Klupp, H. (1975). The pharmacology and toxicology of a new tropane alkaloid derivative. In: The Place of Parasympatholytic Drugs in the Management of Chronic Obstructive Airways Disease. *Postgraduate Medical Journal Suppl.* 7, 51.

Fisher, M. M. (1977). Ketamine in severe bronchospasm. *Anaesthesia* 32, 771.

Friedman, M. and Strang, L. B. (1966). Effect of long-term corticosteroids and corticotrophin on the growth of children. *Lancet* ii, 568.

Gold, M. I. and Helrich, M. (1962). Anesthesia and the asthmatic patient. *Anesthesiology* 23, 149.

Jones, R. S. (1976). *Asthma in Children*. Edward Arnold, London.

Leading article (1973). Analgesics and asthma. *British Medical Journal* 3, 419.

Leading article (1976). Oxygen in bronchial asthma. *British Medical Journal* **1**, 609.

McNeill, R. S. and Ingram, C. G. (1966). Effect of propranolol on ventilatory function. *American Journal of Cardiology* **18**, 473.

Orange, R. P. and Austen, K. F. (1973). Immunologic and pharmacologic receptor control of the release of chemical mediators from human lung. In: *Biological Role of the Immunoglobulin E System*, pp. 151–160. DHEW Publication No. NIH.73–502. Ed. by K. Ishizaka and D. H. Dayton Jr. US Department of Health, Education and Welfare, Public Health Service, National Institutes of Health.

Palmer, K. N. V. and Diament, M. L. (1967). The effect of aerosol isoprenaline on blood gas tensions in severe bronchial asthma. *Lancet* **ii**, 1232.

Palmer, K. N. V. and Kelman, G. R. (1975). Pulmonary function in asthmatic patients in remission. *British Medical Journal* **1**, 485.

Poynter, D. and Spurling, N. W. (1971). Some cardiac effects of beta-adrenergic stimulants in animals. *Postgraduate Medical Journal Suppl.* 47, 21.

Prinkman, L. E. and Whitcomb, F. F. (1959). Decreasing hazards of surgical procedures on patients with asthma. *Diseases of the Chest*, **35**, 35.

Rees, H. A., Borthwick, R. C., Millar, J. S. and Donald, K. W. (1967). Aminophylline in bronchial asthma. *Lancet* **ii**, 1167.

Schnider, S. M. and Papper, E. M. (1961). Anesthesia for the asthmatic. *Anesthesiology* **22**, 886.

Smith, R. H. and Volpitto, P. P. (1960). Bucking and bronchospasm. *Journal of the American Medical Association*. **172**, 1499.

Speizer, R. E., Doll, R. and Heaf, P. (1968). Observations on recent increase in mortality from asthma. *British Medical Journal* **1**, 335.

Weng, T. R. and Levison, H. (1969). Pulmonary function in children with asthma at acute attack and symptom-free status. *American Review of Respiratory Diseases* **99**, 719.

3

Endocrine disorders

Adrenal medulla (phaeochromocytoma)

The condition of phaeochromocytoma was initially described in 1886, and, although Charles Mayo (1927) performed the first successful surgical removal of the tumour, it had not been diagnosed prior to operation. It remained for Pincoffs (1929) to diagnose the condition preoperatively. By 1957, there were over 600 cases recorded in the literature.

The condition is relatively rare and the incidence is believed to be 0·4–2·0 per cent in patients with hypertension. Graham (1951) estimated that in the USA there were 600–800 deaths per year in untreated cases. He also reported a mortality of 25 per cent during surgical removal of a recognized tumour whereas the mortality rose to 50 per cent in operation on patients with unsuspected tumours (Apgar and Papper, 1951).

Phaeochromocytoma is a tumour which secretes an excessive amount of pressor amines. It may arise in the adrenal medulla or in chromaffin tissues elsewhere along the sympathetic chain. The term 'phaeochromocytoma' originally applied to tumours of the adrenal gland which stained brown when treated with chromium. In early life, the neural crest gives rise to the peripheral sympathetic nervous system (the paraganglia) and the adrenal medulla. Paraganglionic cells migrate in close proximity with autonomic ganglion cells and are seen from the base of the skull to the aortic bifurcation. Thus tumours may occur not only in the adrenal gland but anywhere in the sympathetic chain. The tumour may arise in the renal capsule or in the bladder.

It is believed that 10 per cent of all patients with phaeochromocytoma have bilateral tumours and that 10 per cent of these are malignant, the metastases in some cases being capable of secreting amines. There is also an association between neurofibromatosis and phaeochromocytoma. Ganglioneuroma and neuroblastoma are tumours derived from tissues originating in the neural crest and are potentially capable of secreting pressor amines.

Presentation

Patients may present with a history of fainting, headache, vomiting, palpitations, pallor and anxiety. These attacks are often paroxysmal and may be induced by emotional upsets or physical exercise. On examination there are few physical findings, but occasionally a palpable tumour may be present. Pressure on the tumour can induce an attack of hypertension, tachycardia, pallor and sweating. The blood pressure is frequently labile and only raised during the intermittent release of secretions. If the patient presents with hypertension, there is a possibility that there is concomitant myocardial or renal dysfunction. Persistent hypertension may also cause retinal changes. There may be other signs of increased metabolism in addition to anxiety and tachycardia. The condition may be mistaken for thyrotoxicosis, and medullary carcinoma of the thyroid may be present in association with phaeochromocytoma. Glycosuria may occur, suggesting the diagnosis of diabetes.

The undiagnosed patient may present in a bizarre manner as the following examples illustrate. An airline pilot was noted by his colleagues to be agitated and he perspired freely while preparing to land his aircraft. A routine clinical examination revealed no abnormality, but a chest x-ray fortunately included the adrenal area which showed signs of calcification. Further investigation revealed the presence of bilateral phaeochromocytoma. Another patient had been under psychiatric care for depression and was subsequently found to have a phaeochromocytoma.

Some patients may present with normal blood pressure or give a history of attacks of syncope. They may present with hemiplegia. A man aged 74 collapsed while speaking to his neighbour. He was seen afterwards by his doctor to be semiconscious and had a right hemiplegia. The blood pressure was 190/100 mmHg and he was thought to have a subarachnoid haemorrhage. A post-mortem revealed bilateral phaeochromocytoma. In another patient the emotional experience of being admitted to hospital for investigation of phaeochromocytoma was enough to precipitate an attack of hypertension.

Phaeochromocytoma should be suspected in the presence of episodic sustained hypertension, although the diagnosis may be more difficult if the attacks are intermittent or the blood pressure is not raised. Remission is uncommon but Atuk *et al.* (1977) have recorded a case following infarction of the tumour.

Although the diagnosis may be difficult for the physician, the task is even more arduous for the anaesthetist; at operation the complexity of possible causes of labile blood pressure may be difficult to interpret and the decision to proceed with further surgery presents the operating team with a serious dilemma. Ainley-Walker and Woodward (1959) noted during a laminectomy that there was excessive bleeding necessitating the abandonment of the procedure. Further tests revealed the presence of a phaeochromocytoma.

A young woman with papilloedema and a blood pressure of 220/140 mmHg was found to have had a constricted right renal artery on her aortogram. Her blood pressure had been controlled with hexamethonium. At nephrectomy, bleeding was noted to be excessive but when the kidney was removed the blood pressure fell to 60 mmHg. Noradrenaline restored the blood pressure and histological examination of the specimen revealed the presence of phaeochromocytoma.

Less fortunate were the patients who were harbouring the undiagnosed phaeochromocytoma and were operated on for gastric ulcer, gallstones and deflected nasal septum. Although the surgical procedures were successful, pulmonary oedema ensued in the immediate postoperative period and the patients all died. Another patient having varicose veins tied, succumbed when she was turned on her face to carry out the procedure on the back of her legs (personal communications). Seward (1961) recorded a death in the presence of an undiagnosed phaeochromocytoma: a simple cyst in the breast was being removed and the patient died postoperatively.

In obstetric practice, the diagnosis of hypertension may be thought to be due to pre-eclamptic toxaemia. Smith (1973) described three cases, all of whom were delivered by caesarean section; however, one case was undiagnosed prior to surgery and the patient died. Ross et al. (1967), however, reported a case in which attacks occurred only in the postpartum period; it was thought the tumour was compressed when the patient nursed her child.

Phaeochromocytoma also occurs in children. Zintel et al. (1960) found 71 cases in the literature and noted that none survived surgery. Neuroblastoma-secreting pressor amines have also been recorded (Mason et al., 1957) while Smelley and Sandler (1961) described an intrathoracic ganglioneuroma which was secreting catecholamines.

Physiology and pharmacology

Catecholamines* are produced in the adrenal medulla and in the sympathetic nerve terminals. They are formed from phenylalanine which is converted to tyrosine, dopa, dopamine and noradrenaline (Fig. 3.1). In the adrenal medulla the noradrenaline is converted to adrenaline by N-methyltransferase, an enzyme which is absent in the sympathetic nerve ending. It follows, therefore, that tumours arising in the adrenal medulla will secrete predominantly adrenaline whereas tumours arising in extra-adrenal sites will contain mostly noradrenaline.

The adrenaline and noradrenaline are stored in separate cells in the adrenal medulla. When the noradrenaline is released at the nerve terminal, it acts on the receptor site and is taken up again into the nerve terminal. Monoamine oxidase (MAO), which is found in the sympathetic nerve ending, the adrenal medullary cell, liver and kidney, is responsible for the local destruc-

---

* The term catecholamine refers to compounds with a catechol nucleus, i.e. a benzene ring with two hydroxyl groups (a). The introduction of an amine group (b) results in a catecholamine. The common catecholamines are adrenaline, noradrenaline and dopamine.

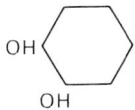

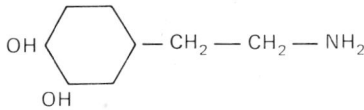

(a)   (b)

L-tyrosine

    ↓ Oxidation

L-dopa

    ↓ Decarboxylation

dopamine

    ↓ Oxidation

noradrenaline

    ↓ Methylation

adrenaline

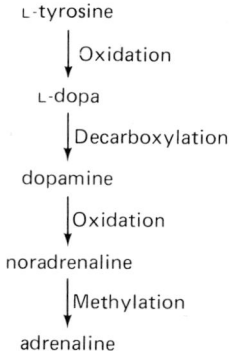

Fig. 3.1   Synthesis of adrenaline.

tion of any pressor amine. Catecholamines which enter the circulation are destroyed by catechol-*O*-methyltransferase (COMT) (Fig. 3.2). Noradrenaline is converted to normetanephrine by COMT and thence by monoamine oxidase (MAO) to 3-methoxy-4-hydroxymandelic aldehyde and finally to 3-methoxy-4-hydroxymandelic acid (vanilmandelic acid or VMA). Some noradrenaline is also converted by MAO to 3,4-dihydroxymandelic acid and this compound is converted by COMT to VMA. Similarly, adrenaline is converted by COMT to metanephrine and oxidized by MAO to 3-methoxy-4-hydroxymandelic aldehyde and finally to VMA. Some adrenaline is acted on by MAO to form 3,4-dihydroxymandelic acid and then converted by COMT to VMA.

The size of the phaeochromocytoma bears no relationship to its ability to produce symptoms. Melmon (1968) divided the tumour into two groups:

Group I. Tumours with a low concentration of catecholamines (under 100 mg) bind the amines poorly and release the catecholamines into the circulation, producing symptoms. The tumour size is often less than 5 g. The turnover of amines is rapid and more metanephrine is produced than VMA.

Group II. The larger tumours with a high catecholamine content (100 mg–10 g) bind the amines well, release only small amounts to the circulation and

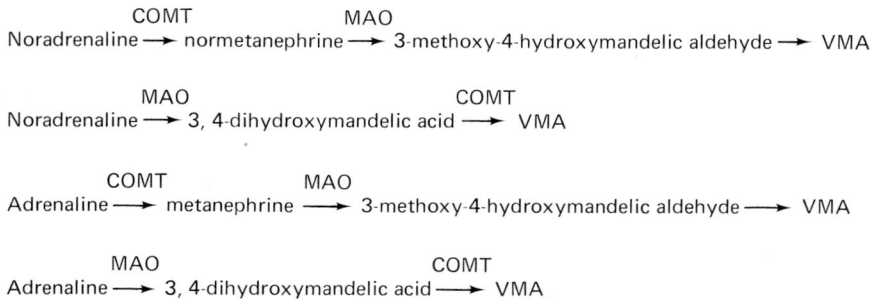

           COMT   MAO
Noradrenaline → normetanephrine → 3-methoxy-4-hydroxymandelic aldehyde → VMA

           MAO   COMT
Noradrenaline → 3,4-dihydroxymandelic acid → VMA

          COMT   MAO
Adrenaline → metanephrine → 3-methoxy-4-hydroxymandelic aldehyde → VMA

        MAO   COMT
Adrenaline → 3,4-dihydroxymandelic acid → VMA

Fig. 3.2   Breakdown pathways of adrenaline and noradrenaline.

only produce symptoms when the gland is large in size. In this situation, the VMA is higher than the metanephrine. There is a close relationship between catecholamines and cyclic AMP which is formed from ATP. Adenyl cyclase activity is increased in the presence of catecholamines. Adenyl cyclase is found in the cell membrane and it is thought that this may be the mediator in the action of catecholamines on the receptor site (second messenger system). Storage of catecholamines is in granules within the vesicle. Daggett and Carruthers (1976) have suggested that the hypertensive crisis due to a phaeochromocytoma is caused by active synthesis of pressor amines rather than release from a stored pool. More recently, Jarrott and Louis (1977) considered that catecholamine production is increased due to excessive synthetic enzymes and that the enzymes involved in their destruction are inhibited.

Alpha and beta receptors

In 1948, Ahlquist proposed the division of adrenergic receptors into alpha (α) and beta (β) groups. The actions of drugs stimulating at the α receptor was exemplified by noradrenaline, and at the β site by isoprenaline. Adrenaline was thought to have combined α and β effects. Ahlquist (1976a, b, 1977) has recently reviewed the present status of α- and β-adrenergic agents. In general, α effects result in stimulation, with the exception of the gut, while β effects are inhibitory, with the exception of the heart. The intestine is inhibited both by α and β effects, the α having a more pronounced effect on the small bowel and the β more on the large bowel. Metabolic effects, such as increasing the blood sugar, are probably mixed effects with the α effect more pronounced in the liver and the β in muscle. Alpha effects cause constriction of vessels in the skin and viscera and increased total peripheral resistance; these result in a rise in blood pressure with reflex slowing of the heart. The intestine is relaxed and the sphincters are constricted. The uterus is stimulated.

Beta receptors are now divided into β1 and β2. The β1 effects are primarily on the heart, resulting in increased heart rate, increased conduction velocity, decreased refractory period and increased contractility. The total peripheral resistance is decreased due to dilation of vessels in the muscles (β2 effect). The bronchi and uterus are relaxed (β2 effect).

Adrenaline has a mixture of α and β effects, with resulting increase in systolic pressure and a fall in diastolic pressure (decreased peripheral resistance). The blood vessels in muscle are dilated but those in the skin and viscera are constricted. The bronchi, intestine and uterus are inhibited. The action of adrenaline on the heart is largely β1.

Phenylephrine has largely α-stimulating effects while isoprenaline has predominantly β effects (β1 and β2). Dopamine acts on the β receptors of the heart. In low doses it increases renal blood flow but in high doses renal vasoconstriction occurs. Isoprenaline has been largely replaced by salbutamol as a β stimulator in the treatment of asthma because of its undesirable β1 side effect, which results in V/Q imbalance and a fall in arterial Po_2.

Diagnosis

The diagnosis of phaeochromocytoma may be elicited from the history, symptoms and physical signs. Palpation of a tumour (palpable tumours are rare) is not recommended, nor are provocation tests using histamine which stimulates the release of catecholamines (Fig. 3.3). Phentolamine has been used to produce a drop in blood pressure and a fall of 35/25 mmHg was said to be diagnostic. The VMA in the urine may be increased and levels above 7 mg per 24 hours (35 μmol) are highly suggestive. VMA random specimens of urine can be related to creatinine levels. Urinary catecholamines are diagnostic at levels of about 200 μg per 24 hours, although in hypertension from other causes the level may rise to 100 μg (normal 20–40 μg per 24 hours). Metanephrine is consistently increased in phaeochromocytoma but is also elevated in other conditions of severe stress; the upper limit of normal is 1 mg per 24 hours (5·5 μmol). Apart from electrocardiographic and x-ray investigations, the tumour may be outlined by retroperitoneal pneumography. Intravenous pyelogram (IVP) may show displacement of the kidney and arteriography may confirm the diagnosis by demonstrating increased vascularity to an adrenal tumour (Fig. 3.4). Vena caval catheterization with measurement of plasma amines may be advantageous in the location of the

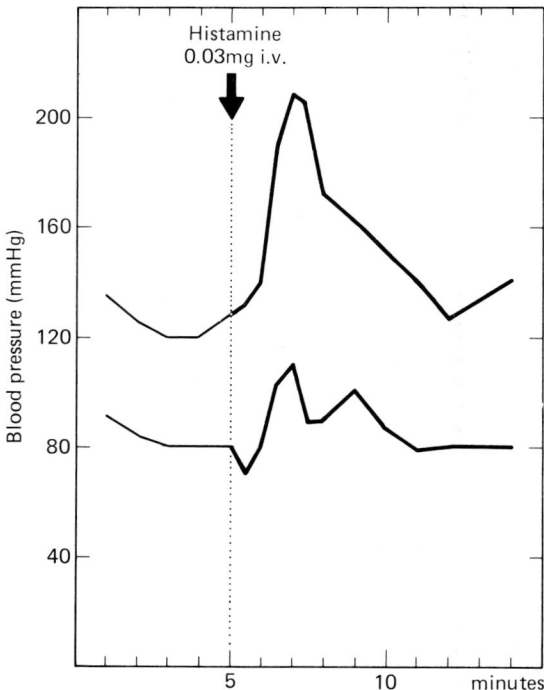

Fig. 3.3   Histamine provocation test, showing dramatic rise in blood pressure.

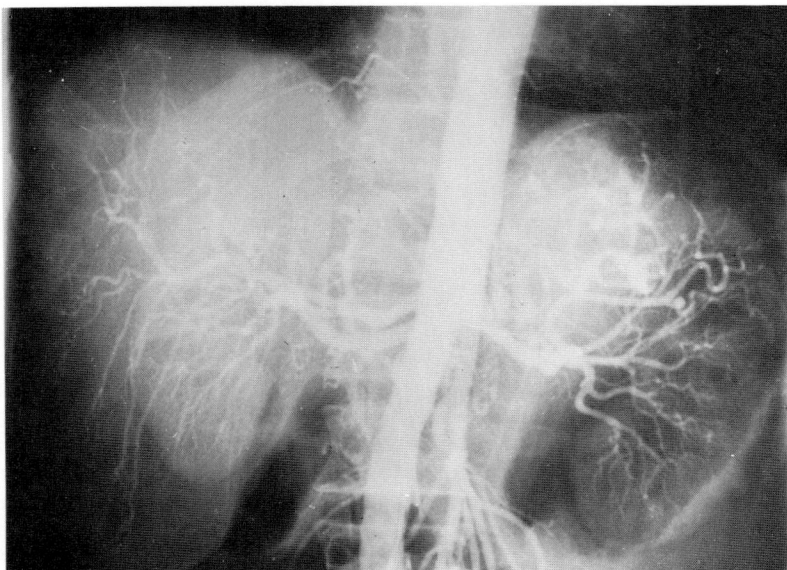

Fig. 3.4 Aortogram, showing outline of phaeochromocytoma in left adrenal gland with increased vascular markings.

tumour site. Levels above $150\,\text{ng}/100\,\text{ml}$ (ng dl^{-1}) are diagnostic (Jiang *et al.*, 1973).

Surgery

The anaesthetist may be confronted with a patient who has phaeochromocytoma in the following circumstances:

(1) elective removal of the tumour;
(2) the arteriogram;
(3) an emergency operation (e.g. appendicectomy);
(4) during an elective procedure such as hernia repair;
(5) pregnancy.

For elective removal of phaeochromocytoma the site of the tumour should be localized, otherwise it may be extremely difficult to find at operation. Manipulation of suspected areas may produce non-specific sympathetic stimulation, particularly in the presence of light anaesthesia. It is helpful to know whether the tumour is bilateral, extremely vascular, malignant, and whether it is in the adrenal gland or an ectopic site.

The fulminating case of an acute attack of phaeochromocytoma may present with cerebral haemorrhage, pulmonary oedema, left ventricular failure and, finally, ventricular fibrillation. Rarely, there have been cases of haemorrhagic necrosis of the tumour following either an attack, in the presence of anticoagulants or after α-adrenergic blockade. At operation the undiagnosed case may present with hypertension, hypotension, arrhythmias and excessive bleeding (Van Way *et al.*, 1976).

Applied pharmacology

Most of the drugs administered in the course of anaesthesia can have an adverse effect on patients with phaeochromocytoma. The management of patients is therefore the result of compromise, selecting those agents with the least possible side effects.

Atropine

Atropine is known to produce tachycardia and possibly increase the cardiac output. Swan (1949) showed that while infusing noradrenaline, atropine caused a more pronounced pressor effect. Barnet *et al.* (1950) also demonstrated that after atropine, noradrenaline initially decreased the pulse rate reflexly, but this was immediately followed by an increased pulse rate and blood pressure. Hyoscine, which has a sedative effect and is a potent antisialogogue, is preferred for premedication. Atropine used prior to neostigmine at the end of the operation always appears to produce tachycardia and hypertension (see Fig. 3.11, p. 82).

Sedation and anaesthesia

Morphine and pethidine are capable of producing hypotension, and morphine is known to release histamine which can precipitate release of catecholamines. Pethidine has recently been reported to have caused hypertension when given intravenously (Lawrence, 1978). Thiopentone can cause myocardial and vasomotor depression, resulting in a fall in blood pressure. This is followed by a compensatory rise in pressure (see Fig. 3.6).

Suxamethonium, although providing ideal conditions for intubation, is considered capable of compressing a tumour by initially increasing muscle tone. Repeated doses may cause muscarinic effects on blood pressure, resulting in hypotension and bradycardia. Large doses of suxamethonium also release histamine. The fasciculations are said to be increased in the presence of high levels of circulating adrenaline and that more suxamethonium is required to produce relaxation. β-Adrenergic-blocking drugs are also thought to potentiate its neuromuscular action. *d*-Tubocurarine produces ganglion blockade and histamine release which can again cause a rise in blood pressure. Gallamine and pancuronium produce tachycardia and may increase the cardiac output.

Chlorpromazine was once considered to be of value for its sedative and adrenergic-blocking properties, but it, too, produces tachycardia. Droperidol has been advocated by Desmonts (Desmonts *et al.*, 1977), and although this has adrenergic-blocking properties, it can produce tachycardia and delayed recovery. Ganglion-blocking drugs potentiate the action of noradrenaline. Geffen and Ross (1956) showed that noradrenaline was potentiated after the injection of hexamethonium. Atropine further potentiated the effect of noradrenaline in the presence of hexamethonium. Similarly, it might be expected that after spinal analgesia the blood pressure would rise when sympathetic tone was abolished in the presence of increased circulating amines. Bromage and Millar (1958) administered epidural blockade for the removal of phaeochromocytoma in a child; during surgery there were rises in blood pressure to 185/125 mmHg, with increased plasma levels of noradrenaline. Bretylium, a drug used in the treatment of hypertension and acting on the postganglionic receptor site, enhances the effect of noradrenaline. Trimetaphan (Arfonad) has been administered to a patient (Case 2, Ross *et al.*, 1967). It caused elevation of the blood pressure and also produced gross cardiac arrhythmias.

Ether releases pressor amines, which often results in tachycardia, but ventricular arrhythmias have seldom been reported. The use of ether has been reported by Schnelle *et al.* (1965). Halothane does not release pressor amines, even in high concentrations. It might be anticipated that squeezing the tumour in the presence of halothane would give rise to ventricular arrhythmias. However, halothane has been used by Rollason (1964) and Murphy *et al.* (1964), and although there were violent fluctuations of blood pressure during the course of surgery, no serious arrhythmias were reported.

Etsten and Shimosato (1965) demonstrated that deep halothane prevented the release of catecholamines. They reported that prior to anaesthesia the plasma level of noradrenaline was 1660 μg/litre and that of adrenaline 2540 μg/litre. The blood pressure was 220/120 mmHg. After the introduction of halothane, the levels dropped to 358 and 326 μg/litre respectively, falling to 69 μg/litre and 35 μg/litre. When the tumour was manipulated, the levels rose to 214 and 57 μg/litre during 0·5 per cent halothane; when 1 per cent halothane was introduced the levels fell to 59 and 29 μg/litre.

Hypoxaemia, CO_2 retention, hypoglycaemia (which may result from an overdose of insulin in the treatment of hyperglycaemia associated with phaeochromocytoma) and blood loss are all capable of releasing catecholamines. Many of the problems associated with anaesthesia for phaeochromocytoma may be due to the fact that modern anaesthesia discourages deep sedation, and this may in itself increase blood levels of pressor amines.

Pharmacology of the adrenoreceptor-blocking drugs

In 1933, Fourneau and Bovet introduced piperoxane (compound 933F) which had a selective depressor effect in phaeochromocytoma. However, it raised the blood pressure in essential hypertension and did not block the effects of infusions of adrenaline and noradrenaline. It remained to Grimson *et al.* to introduce phentolamine (C7337) in 1949.

Phentolamine

Phentolamine (Rogitine) is closely related to tolazoline. In addition to its adrenergic blockade, which is of short duration, it has intrinsic sympathetic activity on the heart, increasing the force of contraction, producing coronary vasodilatation and increasing the heart rate. It has parasympathetic activity, increasing activity of the small intestine, and has a histamine-like action which increases stimulation of gastric secretions and produces vasodilatation. The recommended dose is 0·05–0·1 mg/kg body weight and is often given as a bolus of 2·5–5 mg intravenously.

Phenoxybenzamine

Phenoxybenzamine (Dibenyline) is a β-haloalkylamine. It does not alter or inhibit catecholamines but inhibits the response to circulating noradrenaline by preventing it from penetrating affected cells. The onset of action takes 30–45 minutes because it has to be converted to an ethylenimonium intermediate compound which is active. It is long acting because it forms a covalent bond. Although 50 per cent may be excreted in the first 12 hours and 80 per cent at 24 hours, the duration of action is likely to last up to 30 hours. Small amounts may remain in the body for a week (Nickerson and Collier, 1975). In addition to its α-adrenergic blocking effect, it has antihistamine, antiacetylcholine and anti-5-hydroxytryptamine effects. It produces restlessness, nausea, tachycardia and postural hypotension. It has a soporific effect, and this may be due to a central action on noradrenaline receptors. The persistence of somnolence in the postoperative period may mask the signs of possible cerebral damage due to periods of hypotension or hypertension. It is absorbed poorly by mouth in the dosage of 20–200 mg per day and has to be given intravenously in the order of 0·5–2·0 mg/kg body weight in 250–500 ml dextrose. Patients may complain of stuffy nose and an inability to sweat, and the pupils may be small. It also has a quinidine-like action on the heart.

Indoramin

This is a competitive α-adrenergic-blocking agent which also has antihistamine actions, anti-5-hydroxytryptamine effects and a local analgesic action. It has no antiacetylcholine action but is said to be a cardioinhibitor. It should not be used in conjunction with amine oxidase inhibitors. It is well absorbed and has an immediate effect—the maximum action being in half an hour and lasting up to one hour. It is bound to plasma proteins. The dose recommended is 100 mg q.i.d. (Alps et al., 1972).

α-Adrenergic-blocking drugs, in particular phentolamine, have been known to cause haemorrhagic necrosis of the adrenal gland (Van Way et al., 1976).

β-Adrenergic-blocking drugs

The first β-adrenergic blocking drug to be introduced was dichloroisoprenaline. This drug also had sympathomimetic properties and was too toxic for general use. It also caused a myopathy in the muscle of cats. Pronethalol was next introduced, but was withdrawn because of its tendency to produce carcinoma in animals. This was replaced by propranolol, which is ten times more potent than pronethalol and free of its carcinoma-producing properties.

Propranolol, which is a racemic mixture, is metabolized in the liver to produce metabolites that are active pharmacologically. The dangers of propranolol include bronchospasm in the asthmatic patient, and heart failure in those in whom the heart is dependent on sympathetic drive. It may give rise to hypoglycaemia, especially in diabetics on treatment. It is also recommended that it should be avoided in metabolic acidosis.

Recent additions to the list of β-blocking drugs have included alprenolol, oxprenolol and practolol. Practolol, which is not metabolized, has partial agonistic effects as shown by its intrinsic sympathomimetic effect on heart rate. It has now been found to produce eye and skin complications, plastic peritonitis and pericardial and pleural effusions. Practolol has been withdrawn from long-term medical therapy. In the treatment of phaeochromocytoma, it is essential to avoid the use of a β-adrenergic-blocking drug without the preliminary administration of an α-adrenergic-blocking agent.

Combined α- and β-adrenergic-blocking agent—labetalol

Labetalol has recently been introduced as a drug capable of blocking both α and β adrenoreceptor activity (Farmer et al., 1972). It has a specific action at α and β receptors, both in vivo and in vitro. Intravenously it has a relative potency of α to β antagonist effects of 1:7. It has no partial agonist activity at cardiac β1 receptors and its haemodynamic effects are attributed to its adrenoreceptor blocking actions. Labetalol is less potent than phentolamine or propranolol, and differs from propranolol in decreasing peripheral vascular resistance. It has been used successfully on five occasions for the management of phaeochromocytoma (Rosei et al., 1976), and in one case for the acute hypertension simulating that which occurs in patients with phaeochromocytoma and provoked by clonidine withdrawal. The oral dose may rise to 1600 mg per day but intravenously it seems unnecessary in the anaesthetised patient to give more than 50 mg. The hypotensive effects of labetalol are readily augmented by halothane (Scott et al., 1976) which might be helpful in the management of phaeochromocytoma.

Labetalol may also have a place in the management of the patient in whom the phaeochromocytoma cannot be found and in those with secondary deposits or irremovable tumours. Labetalol withdrawal appears to increase the excretion of catecholamines (Richards, 1976).*

α-Methyl-p-tyrosine

This prevents the hydroxylation of tyrosine to dopa and has been used in the management of phaeochromocytoma (Jones et al., 1968). Although the drug reduces the excretion of catecholamines, it fails to control the blood pressure when the tumour is manipulated at operation. It was suggested that it might have a place in those patients in whom it is unsuitable to use adrenergic-blocking agents for the control of malignant phaeochromocytoma. One of the dangers of its use is that it may cause Parkinsonism.

* More recent work has shown that labetalol does not increase either the plasma noradrenaline or the excretion of pressor amines. It is probable that labetalol or a metabolite interferes with fluorimetric and spectrophotometric methods. VMA excretion is unaffected (Hamilton, Jones et al., 1978).

Management

The management of the patient for the successful removal of a phaeochromo-cytoma depends on the following.

(1) Teamwork between the physician, pharmacologist, surgeon, anaesthetist and nursing staff.

(2) Careful assessment of the patient, with full clinical examination, routine investigations and special investigations.

(3) The blood pressure should be well controlled and any heart failure effectively treated. Diabetes should be treated with insulin as necessary.

(4) Monitoring.

(5) Careful postoperative intensive care.

There is no general agreement on the best anaesthetic technique to be adopted; neither is there a clear relationship between the morbidity and the anaesthetic agent used. The choice of technique, therefore, is usually based on individual experience and preference despite recent advances in the knowledge of pharmacology. The results are often unpredictable as not all cases are alike. There have been extensive reviews of the management, and the following are only a few of these.

Price and Secher (1961) reviewed 26 cases; many of these patients showed violent fluctuations of blood pressure during the operation. Robertson (1962, 1965) reported on the management of 17 patients and the techniques of anaesthesia. He also referred to Griffiths, of the Royal Infirmary, Edinburgh, who used spinal anaesthesia not only to manage the patient at operation but also to confirm the diagnosis when the blood pressure rose due to sympathetic blockade in the presence of a higher level of circulating amines. Bromage and Millar (1958) successfully supervised the patient at operation with epidural analgesia, although there were violent fluctuations of blood pressure.

In 1964, Gifford *et al.* reviewed 76 cases from the Mayo Clinic. The anaesthetic management was discussed by Schnelle *et al.* (1965); they comment on the problems associated with sustained hypertension and intermittent hypertension, and that blood pressure rose as the expression of the exaggerated response to surgical stimuli during light anaesthesia and during squeezing of the tumour. All the deaths were in the group with sustained hypertension. The agents used were ether, tubocurarine, phentolamine and vasopressors. In one of the patients in whom halothane was used, cardiac arrest developed when the tumour was being palpated.

In 1966, De Blasi reviewed the management of anaesthesia and the use of α- and β-blocking drugs. Ross *et al.* (1967) reported on the detailed management of 27 patients with phaeochromocytoma, operated on, on 30 occasions. They traced the development of α- and β-adrenergic-blocking drugs in controlling possible hypertensive crisis following the induction of anaesthesia, avoiding the extreme fluctuations of blood pressure during manipulation of the tumour at operation and the sudden hypotension which immediately followed removal of the tumour. Techniques were adopted to prevent the sudden release of large concentrations of catecholamines with the possible sensitization of the myocardium, which could produce arrhythmias in the presence of certain anaesthetic agents. It was noted that complications were more prevalent in patients with sustained hypertension. Ross *et al.* outlined the management of blood pressure before and during operation and after removal of the tumour. They commented on the control of tachycardia, the hazards of anaesthetic agents, the prevention of arrhythmias, the effects of hypercapnia, haemorrhage and adrenocortical insufficiency, and outlined a detailed programme for the preoperative management (see p. 74). Gitlow *et al.* (1971) presented a review of the management, commenting on the use of phenoxybenzamine and α-amino-p-tyrosine and found there was no need to use β-adrenergic-blocking drugs. Katz and Wolf (1971) discussed the use of nitroprusside and suggested that there was no need for complicated regimens of adrenergic blockage: possible peaks in blood pressure could be easily controlled by nitroprusside.

Coeliac plexus blockade has been advocated prior to surgery, but this involves turning the patient on to one side and the possibility of inducing an attack; nevertheless, correctly performed, the blockade has proved to be advantageous (personal communication).

Van Way *et al.* (1974) presented a detailed review of phaeochromocytoma, including the history, anatomy, embryology, physiology, pharmacology, genetics, pathology, clinical aspects and management. They reviewed the results of 138 cases treated surgically at the Mayo Clinic; there were 4 deaths due to uncontrolled haemorrhage and 2 to cardiac arrest at operation. After 1965, when adrenergic blocking agents became available, there were no deaths in this series.

Stamenkovic and Spierdijk (1976) reported on the management of 12 patients using α- and β-blocking drugs and anaesthesia consisting of droperidol, fentanyl, nitrous oxide, oxygen and pancuronium. They used sodium nitroprusside at operation to control the blood pressure. There are no details or charts of the blood pressure changes at operation, and it appears that they only used nitroprusside in their last five cases.

Desmonts *et al.* (1977) reviewed 102 cases of phaeochromocytoma. In 14 patients they used thiopentone, tubocurarine and a narcotic, and hypertensive crises were treated with phentolamine; trimetaphan was used on three occasions, causing serious cardiac arrhythmias. Noradrenaline infusions were required in this group. In a second group, of 50 patients, anaesthesia consisted of thiopentone, suxamethonium or pancuronium, and halothane. Noradrenaline was also used in these patients. In a third group, of 30 patients, anaesthesia was induced with droperidol and phenoperidine, followed by thiopentone and pancuronium; hypertensive crises were treated with phentolamine and nitroprusside. Lignocaine was used for the treatment of arrhythmias. No adrenergic-blocking drugs were used. No attempt was made to classify the severity of the hypertension in these patients. In the droperidol group, the systolic blood pressure was stable but at high values, often greater than 250 mmHg.

Management of the patient for elective surgery

This regimen follows that laid down by Ross *et al.* (1967). They held the view that violent swings of blood pressure during operation are undesirable because of possible cardiovascular and neurological complications. With the advent of adrenergic-blocking agents, fluctuations in blood pressure were minimized and the use of noradrenaline following removal of the tumour was unnecessary.

Harrison, Bartlett and Seaton (1968) reviewed the indications for α-adrenergic blockade:

(1) a blood pressure greater than 200/130 mmHg;
(2) frequent severe uncontrolled hypertensive attacks;
(3) use of β-adrenergic blockers;
(4) a haematocrit greater than 50 per cent.

Indications for β-adrenergic blockade included:

(1) a pulse rate greater than 140 per minute;
(2) any history of arrhythmia;
(3) persistent ventricular ectopic beats;
(4) pure adrenaline-secreting tumours.

While awaiting operation, hypertension is controlled with oral phenoxybenzamine, and any tachycardia with oral propranolol. Three days prior to operation, the patient is given phenoxybenzamine intravenously in the dose of 0·5–2 mg/kg body weight (average 1 mg) in 250 ml of 5 per cent dextrose over a period of $\frac{1}{2}$–1 hour. Postural hypotension will ensue unless the patient is kept in bed. The patient's pulse rate and blood pressure are monitored throughout the infusion. This is repeated for three days and propranolol 40 mg is administered by mouth if the pulse rate rises above 80 per minute. For the average adult, papaveretum 15 mg and 0·3 mg hyoscine are used for premedication, and blood pressure and pulse rate are monitored from that period onwards. Before induction of anaesthesia, arterial and central venous cannulation is performed to allow direct monitoring of these pressures. The radial artery may be difficult to palpate as an adrenergic paroxysm can readily constrict the vessel. The e.c.g. and heart rate are monitored continuously. A catheter is inserted to measure urinary output. Measurement of cardiac output is unlikely to be performed in the routine management, but Darby and Prys-Roberts (1976) were able to monitor the pulmonary artery and pulmonary capillary wedge pressures (PCWP) by means of a Swan–Ganz catheter in a patient who was found at operation to have a phaeochromocytoma. During periods of hypertension, the pulmonary capillary wedge pressure rose to 24 mmHg, suggesting severe strain on the left side of the heart. A diagnosis of phaeochromocytoma was made when 5 mg of phentolamine reduced the blood pressure markedly while the PCWP fell to 8 mmHg. If the blood pressure is labile on the morning of the operation, phenoxybenzamine may be required; because there is a delay before it is effective, it is necessary to administer it early. Two intravenous infusions are established. The following drugs should be available during operation: phentolamine, phenoxybenzamine, isoprenaline, noradrenaline and hydrocortisone. Phenoxybenzamine potentiates the sedative effects of morphine and it is unnecessary to use more than 100–200 mg thiopentone. Thiopentone is administered slowly and intubation performed with the aid of suxamethonium. The intubation period should be as short as possible to avoid unnecessary fluctuations of blood pressure due to hypoxia. Anaesthesia is maintained with nitrous oxide, oxygen and intermittent tubocurarine and fentanyl. The blood pressure may fluctuate during induction, during intubation, during positioning of the patient on the operating table, during surgical manipulation of the tumour and when the blood supply to the tumour is ligated. Hypertensive episodes are marked by rises in blood pressure and CVP. It must always be remembered that there may be a second tumour secreting pressor amines. If the tumour has not been located preoperatively, it is seldom found at operation. Incomplete α blockade may aid in the diagnosis by allowing greater fluctuations of the blood pressure during stimulation in suspected areas, but these are often the result of non-specific surgical stimulation during light anaesthesia. Such a test should always be performed when anaesthesia has been supplemented by further doses of tubocurarine or fentanyl. If bleeding is profuse, whole blood and crystalloids will be necessary to make up for the loss. It would be advisable to have ten units of blood available and to administer these through a blood warmer and a microfilter. Haemorrhage is a particular hazard in the presence of α blockade. When β blockade is significant, the pulse rate will not increase in response to a haemorrhage. At the end of the operation, atropine and neostigmine are administered to reverse the neuromuscular blockade; after atropine there is always a substantial rise in blood pressure. Naloxone may be necessary to antagonise the respiratory depression of the fentanyl.

Postoperatively, the patient is carefully monitored for at least 24 hours as there may still be circulating amines which may cause arrhythmias. If bilateral adrenal tumours have been removed, steroids will be necessary. α-Adrenergic blocking drugs such as phenoxybenzamine are long acting and their effects persist into the postoperative period, causing not only postural hypotension but also somnolence and ileus. They may mask the signs of possible cerebral damage resulting from periods of hypotension or hypertension. Care is necessary with β-adrenergic-blocking drugs such as propranolol which potentiate the action of drugs used in the treatment of diabetes. An unusual complication reported recently with propranolol has been the presence of non-ketotic hyperosmolar diabetic coma (Podolsky and Pattavina, 1973).

Hazards in the first 72 hours following surgery

(1) *Haemorrhage*. The effects of haemorrhage in the patient during the postoperative period may be difficult to interpret because of the persistence of the effect of adrenergic blockers. There is a possible danger of even overtransfusion.

(2) *Adrenal failure* may occur, especially if the tumour is bilateral or the

opposite adrenal gland has become infarcted during handling. Use of intravenous hydrocortisone may be necessary.

(3) There may be a *second tumour* which secretes catecholamines. Interpretation of the effects of haemorrhage in the presence of a second secreting tumour is extremely difficult.

(4) *Low blood volume*. This may be due to inadequate transfusion at operation, or the loss of fluids as may occur in postoperative ileus. The suggestion by Brunjes, Johns and Crane (1960) that in phaeochromocytoma there is a reduced circulating blood volume has not been confirmed by others (Sjoerdsma *et al.*, 1966) nor in the present series.

(5) *Persistent effect of adrenergic blockers*. These may cause postural hypotension, even without any fluid loss. Labetalol seems to offer advantages over coventional drugs, as it is less liable to produce this effect.

(6) *Cardiomyopathy*. Fauvre *et al.* (1972) reported that cardiomyopathy occurred in 58 per cent of cases. There are said to be multifocal myocardial lesions described as myofibrillar degeneration and thought to be due to the high concentration of pressor amines (Szakacs and Mehlman, 1960). Damage to cardiac muscle appears to be present in those patients with phaeochromocytoma who are untreated. Bagnall *et al.* (1976) have advocated the use of α-methyl-p-tyrosine in the management of myocarditis.

(7) *Renal damage*. Kidney damage may be due to persistent hypertension (Leather *et al.*, 1962), although there may be coexisting renal artery stenosis, possibly due to the effect of pressor amines (Van Way *et al.*, 1970). Acute tubular necrosis may result from a period of hypotension at the operation.

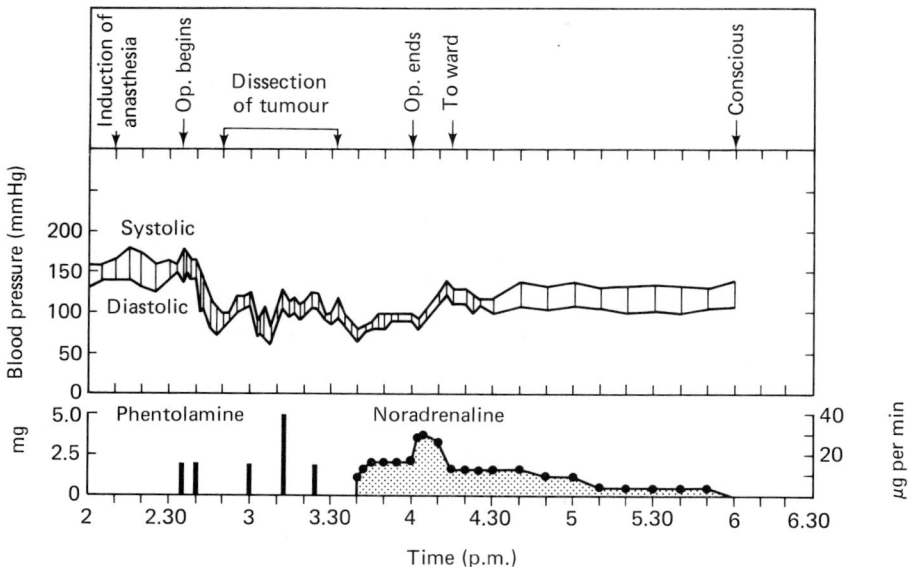

Fig. 3.5 Phaeochromocytoma; case 1. Use of phentolamine and noradrenaline.

(8) *Hypotension* in the postoperative period is reputed to be due to the reduction of pressor amines from previous high concentrations.

(9) *Diabetes*. It must not be forgotten that patients with diabetes associated with phaeochromocytoma still require to have their blood sugar monitored regularly, as their insulin requirements may alter once the tumour is removed. Hypoglycaemia is rapid in onset whereas hyperglycaemic coma takes longer to develop. β-Adrenergic-blocking drugs potentiate the action of oral anti-diabetic drugs and insulin.

In the review of the patients reported by Ross *et al.* (1967) there were 27 patients operated on and 3 deaths. One death was associated with massive haemorrhage in the presence of β blockade; one died from septicaemia, infection having gained entry at the site of one of the monitoring lines; and one had a large retroperitoneal haematoma. To date, the same unit has operated on another 33 cases with only 1 death attributed to over-transfusion.

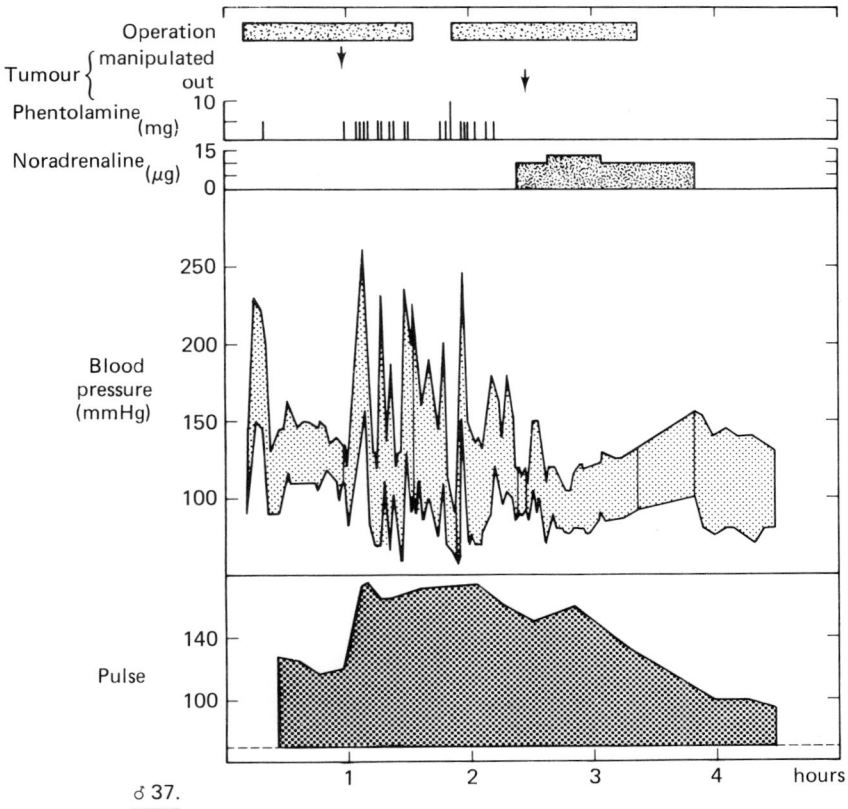

Fig. 3.6 Phaeochromocytoma; case 2. Use of phentolamine and noradrenaline. Note extreme rise in blood pressure following induction.

The following case reports illustrate some of the problems in the operative management of phaeochromocytoma and trace the development of the use of adrenergic-blocking agents.

Case 1. A 23-year-old housewife, with a four-year history of sweating, palpitations, headaches and heart failure, was 20 weeks' pregnant on admission and had a malignant hypertension with a blood pressure of 230/140 mmHg and a pulse rate of 120. At operation (Fig. 3.5) the blood pressure was under reasonable control, but on removal of the tumour the blood pressure fell to 80/60 mmHg, requiring a noradrenaline infusion for $2\frac{1}{2}$ hours after operation. Fourteen hours postoperatively, the blood pressure fell to 90/70 mmHg and the pulse rate rose to 140. Despite blood transfusion and noradrenaline, the blood pressure continued to fall. At a further operation a retroperitoneal haematoma was found, resulting from a dislodged ligature on the adrenal vein. Another phaeochromocytoma was found in the other gland. The patient died.

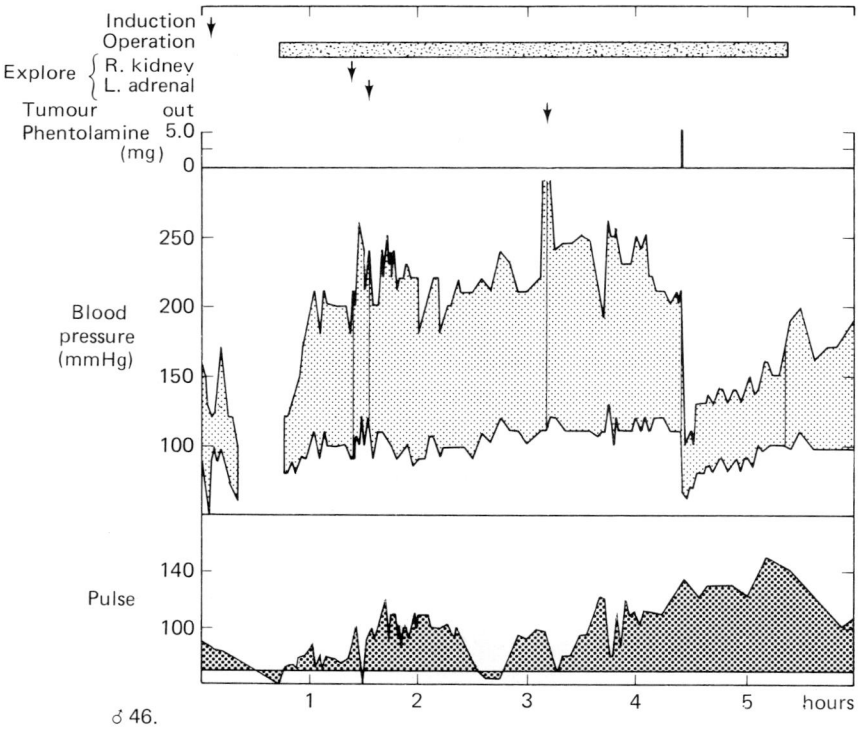

Fig. 3.7   Phaeochromocytoma; case 2. Preparation with phenoxybenzamine and pronethalol (second operation). Use of phentolamine as test dose to see if more tumours present.

Case 2. This patient was a 37-year-old company director who had a large phaeochromocytoma removed from his right adrenal gland. No special preparation of the patient was undertaken and during the operation there were wide fluctuations of blood pressure, on occasion reaching to 250/150 mmHg and the pulse over 150 per minute. The surgical procedure had to be stopped for half an hour on one occasion until the blood pressure could be controlled (Fig. 3.6).

Nine years later, the symptoms recurred and he was prepared for operation with phenoxybenzamine 60 mg daily orally and pronetholol 100 mg t.d.s. As the second tumour could not be located pre-operatively he was deliberately underdosed with phenoxybenzamine. Because of this, there were peaks of blood pressure at operation (Fig. 3.7) but the pulse rate was well controlled. After the tumour was removed, the systolic blood pressure was still over 200 mmHg. A challenging dose of phentolamine was given to test for any tumour still present and this resulted in a marked fall in blood pressure to 90/60 mmHg with an increased pulse rate. This patient still has further tumours present and is controlled with 10 mg phenoxybenzamine and 40 mg propranolol by mouth five times a day.

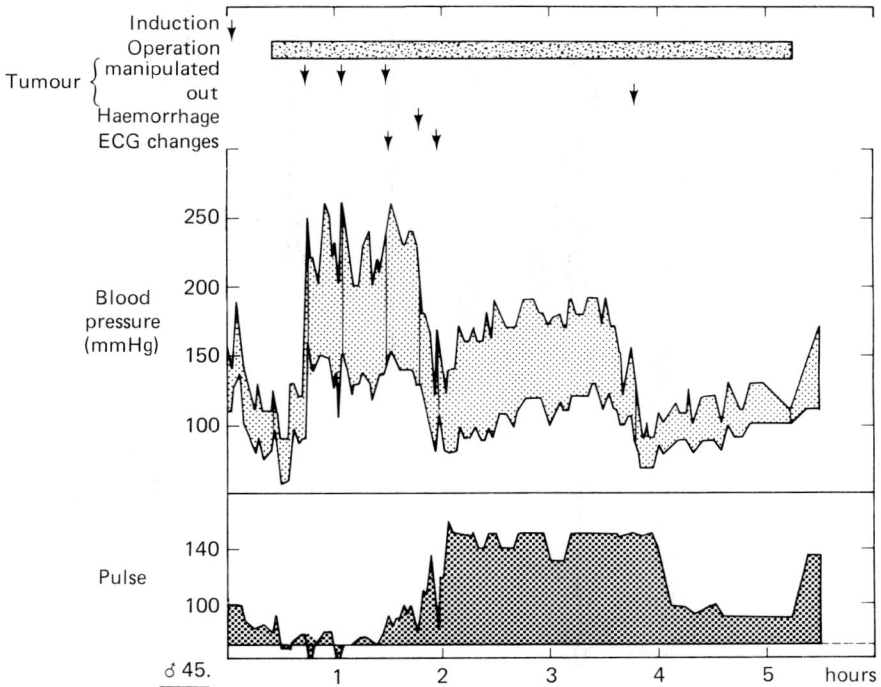

Fig. 3.8 Phaeochromocytoma; case 3. Preparation with phenoxybenzamine and propranolol. Pulse rate well controlled until haemorrhage ensued.

Case 3. A 45-year-old civil servant with a history of palpitations, sweating and tightness of the chest was prepared for operation with phenoxybenzamine 80 mg and propranolol 40 mg orally for three days before the operation. During manipulation of the tumour the blood pressure rose to 250/150 mmHg but there was little change in the pulse rate even though this was an adrenaline-producing tumour. During a period of brisk haemorrhage the blood pressure fell to 110/70 mmHg, the pulse rate rose to 150 per minute and was accompanied by frequent extrasystoles and left bundle branch block. This disappeared following the rapid transfusion of three units of blood. When the tumour was removed, the pressure fell to 90/70 mmHg and rose to 110/80 mmHg with the transfusion of a further unit of blood. Noradrenaline was not required (Fig. 3.8).

Case 4. A 17-year-old boy was found to have a blood pressure of 210/150 mmHg and a pulse rate of 124 per minute at a routine medical examina-

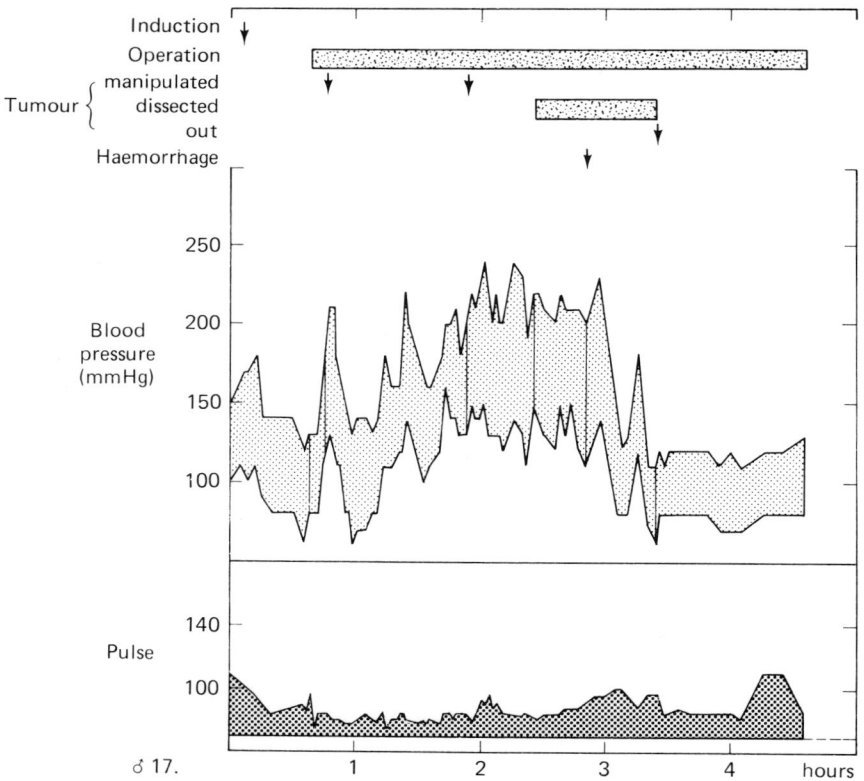

Fig. 3.9 Phaeochromocytoma; case 4. Preparation with phenoxybenzamine and pronethalol. Beta blockade prevented the tachycardia associated with haemorrhage.

tion. He was prepared for surgery with 50 mg phenoxybenzamine and 100 mg pronethanol by mouth for three days before the operation. At operation, there were fluctuations of blood pressure which confirmed that the oral phenoxybenzamine was inadequate in the preparation of patients. During surgery, when there was a period of brisk haemorrhage, the pulse remained remarkably steady, possibly due to the fact that the tumour, which was extra-adrenal, was secreting only noradrenaline. In these circumstances, the presence of β blockade may mask the tachycardia of haemorrhage (Fig. 3.9).

Case 5. A 12-year-old schoolgirl complained of nausea and sweating. Her blood pressure was 210/150 mmHg. She was prepared for operation with oral phenoxybenzamine and with 50 mg given intravenously prior to surgery. Propranolol was given in the dose of 40 mg t.d.s. There were violent swings of blood pressure due to the inadequate preparation with phenoxybenzamine but the pulse rate was reasonably well controlled by propranolol at operation (Fig. 3.10).

Case 6. This was a patient aged 54 who had been treated for heart failure with digoxin and diuretics. She was found to be hypertensive with a blood pressure of 170/100 mmHg. The patient was prepared for surgery with

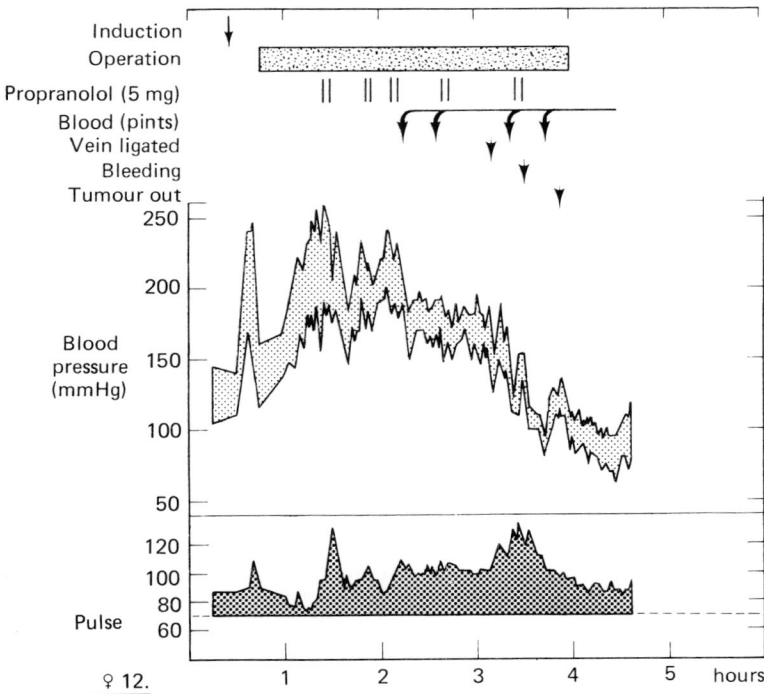

Fig. 3.10   Phaeochromocytoma; case 5. Inadequate preparation with phenoxybenzamine.

phenoxybenzamine 50 mg intravenously for three days and oral practolol. An adrenal tumour was removed and there was remarkably good control of blood pressure and pulse rate during operation (Fig. 3.11).

The examples above show that with careful and correct doses of α- and β-blocking drugs, the control of blood pressure and pulse rate at operation is satisfactory. These adrenergic-blocking drugs impose potential hazards on the patient and there is need for careful monitoring and interpretation of the results. Phenoxybenzamine results in the patient being very drowsy after operation but apparently it can also enhance the ability of red cells to offload oxygen (Watkins et al., 1976). There have been cases where, after the successful removal of a solitary tumour, there have been episodes of cardiac arrhythmias. The use of blocking drugs, however, has resulted in a reduction in the use of noradrenaline, with its attendant dangers—such as difficulty in weaning the patient from the vasopressor, the adjustment of the dose and the risk of extravasation at the site of the intravenous infusion with resultant skin necrosis.

Rosei et al. (1976) reported on the use of labetalol in five patients with phaeochromocytoma. In four of the five patients the blood pressure was satisfactorily controlled and it was used on two occasions prior to surgery. In

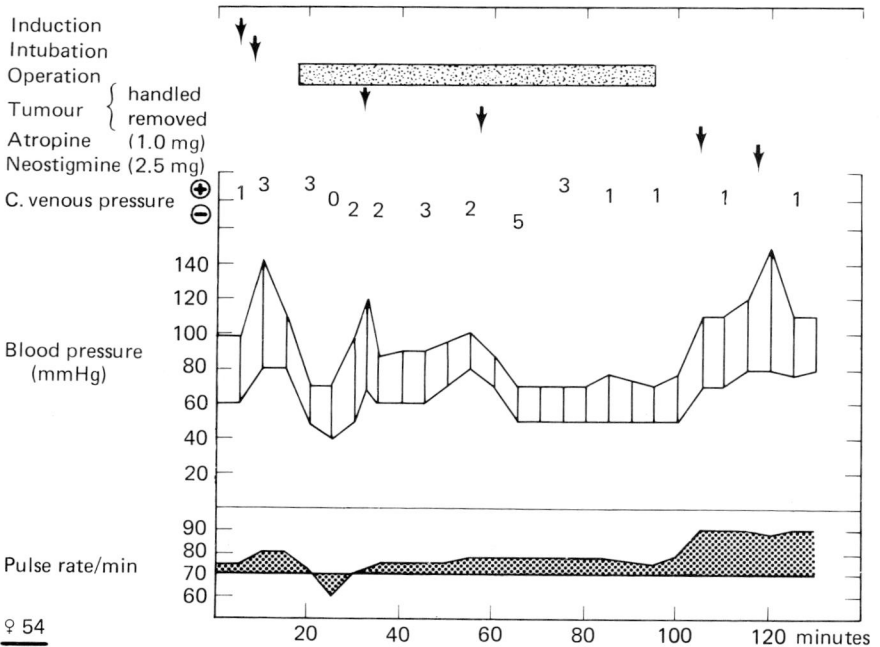

Fig. 3.11   Phaeochromocytoma; case 6. Preparation with phenoxybenzamine and practolol. Good control of blood pressure and pulse rate. Note rise in blood pressure and pulse rate after intravenous atropine.

one patient it was impossible to suppress the attacks of hypertension, and at operation propranolol and phenoxybenzamine were also ineffectual.

Case 7. (Fig. 3.12) An electronics engineer aged 50 had had a phaeochromocytoma removed two years previously at a hospital abroad and on further investigation was found to have a tumour in the opposite adrenal gland. His blood pressure was 170/120 mmHg and he was stabilized with 400 mg labetalol t.d.s. which brought it down to 130/90 mmHg. The blood pressure, pulse rate and central venous pressure were remarkably stable during surgery. Early in the operation the blood pressure rose to over 200 mmHg, which was thought to be due to too light anaesthesia. The blood pressure fell to 150 mmHg after fentanyl had been administered A further rise in blood pressure and pulse rate was controlled with two doses of labetalol 25 mg intravenously and from then on no peaks of blood pressure or pulse rate

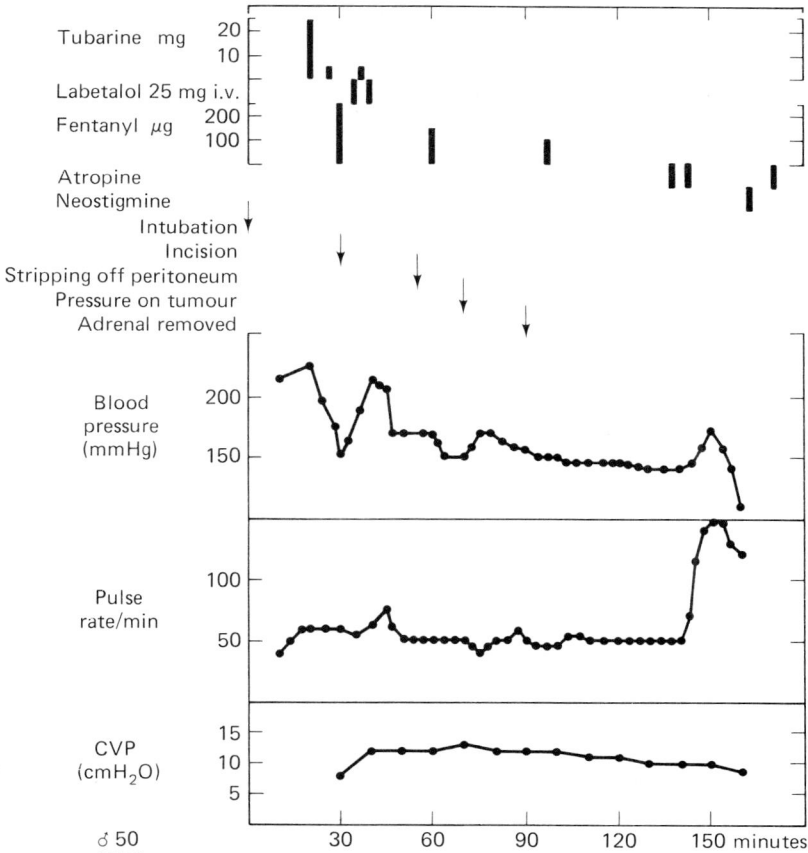

Fig. 3.12 Phaeochromocytoma; case 7. Preparation with labetalol. Good control of blood pressure and pulse rate.

occurred. At the end of operation the blood pressure and pulse rate rose with the administration of atropine prior to the neostigmine. The management of this patient during surgery was remarkably uneventful compared with the previous cases with or without α- and β-blocking drugs. There was no drowsiness as is seen with phenoxybenzamine. The nursing staff in the intensive care unit expressed surprise that, as the patient seemed so well, he should be sent to their care! Labetalol in this one patient appears to be a distinct improvement on previous therapy, although with a ratio of β to α blockade of 7:1 it might have been expected that the blood pressure would have been more labile.

Phaeochromocytoma and pregnancy

Fortunately, this combination is rare, although there have been numerous reports in the literature (Gemmell, 1955; Brenner et al., 1972; Brusanowski et al., 1972; Smith, 1973; Leake et al., 1977). All authors agree that the risks to the mother and child are greatly increased during pregnancy. Van Way et al. (1974) recorded two patients who had unsuspected phaeochromocytoma in pregnancy. In one, profound hypertension developed after delivery; six months later a diagnosis of phaeochromocytoma was made and the tumour successfully removed. In the other patient, ventricular fibrillation developed during an emergency operation for a ruptured ectopic pregnancy and the tumour was only discovered at post-mortem. Smith (1973) reported three cases, one of which was diagnosed at post-mortem.

Case 8. A 27-year-old in her second pregnancy was found to have a history of headache and a blood pressure of 220/130 mmHg. She had given a history of headaches since the age of 16 and at the age of 25, during her first pregnancy, she had developed hypertension. She was delivered at that time by caesarean section (performed after 32 weeks' gestation) and convalescence was stormy. On this occasion her urinary VMA was 10 mg per 24 hours (normal 1·8–7·0), metanephrine 3·8 mg (1·3) and the noradrenaline 547 μg (10–70). She was treated with phenoxybenzamine 10 mg t.d.s., which lowered the pressure to 150/100 mmHg. Though Van Way et al. (1974) have advocated the simultaneous delivery of the child by caesarean section and removal of the tumour, it was felt on this occasion that only caesarean section should be performed. Although phenoxybenzamine is highly lipid soluble at body pH, it appears to cause little effect on the fetus. On the day before operation, the patient was given 65 mg of phenoxybenzamine intravenously, and anaesthesia on this occasion consisted of thiopentone; suxamethonium was used to provide relaxation for intubation, and anaesthesia was maintained with nitrous oxide, oxygen and 0·5 per cent halothane; 7 mg decamethonium was used for muscle relaxation. Anaesthesia was uneventful save a few ectopic beats during light anaesthesia at the end of the operation. Decamethonium was chosen to avoid the need for atropine and neostigmine to reverse a non-depolarizing block at the end of operation. Ergometrine was avoided and two units of oxytocin were given slowly intravenously (Fig. 3.13).

Six weeks after surgery was performed, the patient had an aortogram under phenoxybenzamine cover; it revealed a tumour at the aortic bifurcation and an aberrant right renal artery which went to the lower pole of the right kidney; it also showed that the tumour received its blood supply from a branch of the left common iliac and the lower lumbar and median sacral arteries. At a subsequent operation under phenoxybenzamine and practolol cover, the tumour, which was extra-adrenal, was removed with minimal disturbance to blood pressure and pulse rate.

Fulminating attack of hypertension

During a fulminating attack, it is essential initially to infuse phentolamine to obtain immediate control of the blood pressure and phenoxybenzamine to provide a prolonged effect. If the blood pressure is adequately controlled, arrangements can be made to verify the position of the possible tumour. Failure to control the blood pressure may result in an attack of pulmonary

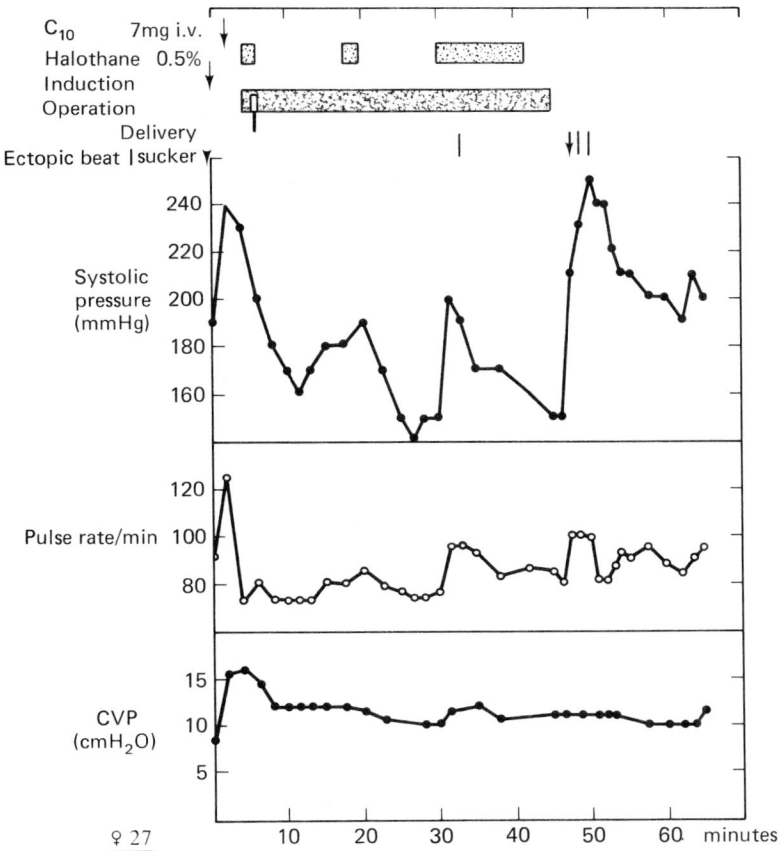

Fig. 3.13 Phaeochromocytoma; case 8. Caesarean section in the presence of phaeochromocytoma.

oedema, cerebral haemorrhage, ventricular tachycardia and fibrillation and hyperpyrexia. Labetalol has been shown to be of value during an attack (personal observation).

The unpredicted phaeochromocytoma

If there is unexplained hypertension and cardiac arrhythmias during an operation then the possibility of a phaeochromocytoma should be considered. It is essential to administer an α-adrenergic-blocking drug first, as a β blocker given alone will cause the blood pressure to rise even higher. If bleeding is profuse, surgery may have to be abandoned and investigations undertaken to confirm the diagnosis. Labetalol may have a place in the management of the undiagnosed phaeochromocytoma occurring unexpectedly during surgery.

The aortogram

The aortogram is often a more hazardous procedure than the actual operation for the removal of the tumour. The investigation is carried out in the x-ray department where the lighting may be subdued and the monitoring facilities meagre compared with that available for the definitive surgery. The danger periods are the same as those described for the operation. In addition, there is the risk that the injection of the dye may precipitate an attack. Alpha- and β-adrenergic-blocking drugs should be readily available. On no account should ganglion-blocking drugs be administered in order to reduce blood flow to produce better x-ray pictures.

Although opinions may vary as to the best techniques of anaesthesia for phaeochromocytoma and the decision whether to use adrenergic-blocking drugs or not, the successful management of the patient depends on careful monitoring and the use of drugs and techniques which are familiar to the anaesthetist. Each drug and technique has its advantages and disadvantages.

References

Ahlquist, R. P. (1976a). The adrenergic receptor. *American Heart Journal* **92**, 661.

Ahlquist, R. P. (1976b). The adrenergic blocking agent. *American Heart Journal* **92**, 804.

Ahlquist, R. P. (1977). The beta blocking agents. *American Heart Journal* **93**, 117.

Ainley-Walker, J. C. S. and Woodward, J. W. (1959). Acute hypertension developing under anaesthesia; a near fatality. *British Journal of Anaesthesia* **31**, 167.

Alps, B. J., Hill, M. *et al.* (1972). Quantitative analysis on isolated organs of the autonomic blocking properties of indoramin hydrochloride. *British Journal of Pharmacology* **44**, 52.

Apgar, V. and Papper, E. M. (1951). Phaeochromocytoma: anesthetic management during surgical treatment. *Archives of Surgery* **62**, 634.

Atuk, N. O., Teja, A. K. *et al.* (1977). Avascular necrosis of phaeochromocytoma followed by spontaneous remission. *Archives of Internal Medicine* **137**, 1073.

Bagnall, W. E., Salway, G. J. *et al.* (1976). Phaeochromocytoma with myocarditis, managed with α-methyl-para-tyrosine. *Postgraduate Medical Journal* **52**, 653.

Barnet, A. J., Blacket, P. B. *et al.* (1950). Action of noradrenaline in man and its relation to phaeochromocytoma and hypertension. *Clinical Science* **9**, 151.

Brenner, W. I., Yen, S. S. C. *et al.* (1972). Phaeochromocytoma—serial studies during pregnancy. *American Journal of Obstetrics and Gynecology* **113**, 778.

Bromage, P. R. and Millar, R. A. (1958). Epidural blockade and circulating catecholamine levels in a child with phaeochromocytoma. *Canadian Anaesthetists' Society Journal* **5**, 282.

Brunjes, S., Johns, V. J. and Crane, M. G. (1960). Phaeochromocytoma: postoperative shock and blood volume. *New England Journal of Medicine* **262**, 393.

Brusanowski, Z. Z., Jorgenson, E. O. *et al.* (1972). Phaeochromocytoma in obstetric practice. *Obstetrics and Gynecology* **22**, 120.

Daggett, P. and Carruthers, M. (1976). Integrated concentrations of catecholamines in phaeochromocytoma. *Lancet* **ii**, 830.

Darby, E. and Prys-Roberts, C. (1976). Unusual presentation of phaeochromocytoma—management of anaesthesia and cardiovascular monitoring. *Anaesthesia* **31**, 913.

De Blasi, S. (1966). The management of the patient with a phaeochromocytoma. *British Journal of Anaesthesia* **38**, 740.

Desmonts, J. M., Le Houelleur, J., Redmond, P. and Duvaildestin, P. (1977). Anaesthetic management of patients with a phaeochromocytoma—a review of 102 cases. *British Journal of Anaesthesia* **49**, 991.

Dornhurst, A. C. and Laurence, D. R. (1963). Use of pronethalol in phaeochrome tumours. *British Medical Journal* **2**, 1250.

Etsten, B. E. and Shimosato, S. (1965). Halothane anesthesia and catecholamine levels in a patient with phaeochromocytoma. *Anesthesiology* **26**, 688.

Farmer, J. B., Kennedy, L. *et al.* (1972). Pharmacology of AH 5158; a drug which blocks both α- and β-adrenoceptors. *British Journal of Pharmacology* **45**, 660.

Fauvre, F. M., John, D. *et al.* (1972). Cardiomyopathy due to phaeochromocytoma. *California Medicine* **117**, 58.

Fourneau, E. and Bovet, D. (1933). Recherches sur l'action sympathicolytique d'un nouveau dérivé du dioxane. *Archives internationales de Pharmacodynamie et de Therapie* **46**, 178.

Geffen, T. J. B. and Ross, E. J. (1956). Potentiation of pressor effect of noradrenaline by hexamethonium in man. *Clinical Science* **15**, 271.

Gemmell, A. A. (1955). Phaeochromocytoma and the obstetrician. *Journal of Obstetrics and Gynaecology of the British Commonwealth* **62**, 125.
Gifford, R. W., Kvale, W. F. *et al.* (1964). Clinical features, diagnosis and treatment of phaeochromocytoma. *Mayo Clinic Proceedings* **39**, 281.
Gitlow, S. E., Pertsemlidis, D. *et al.* (1971). Management of patients with phaeochromocytoma. *American Heart Journal* **82**, 557.
Graham, J. B. (1951). Phaeochromocytoma and hypertension. *Surgery, Gynecology and Obstetrics* **92**, 105.
Grimson, K. S., Longing, F. M. *et al.* (1949). Treatment of a patient with phaeochromocytoma. Use of an adrenolytic drug before and during operation. *Journal of the American Medical Association* **140**, 1273.
Hamilton, C. A., Jones, D. H. *et al.* (1978). Does labetolol increase excretion of urinary catecholamines? *British Medical Journal* **2**, 800.
Harrison, T. S., Bartlett, J. D. Jr. and Seaton, J. F. (1968). Current evaluation and management of phaeochromocytoma. *Annals of Surgery* **168**, 701.
Jarrott, B. and Louis, W. J. (1977). Abnormality in enzymes involved in catecholamine synthesis and metabolism in phaeochromocytoma. *Clinical Science and Molecular Medicine* **53**, 529.
Jiang, N., Stoffer, S. S. *et al.* (1973). Laboratory and clinical observations with a two-column plasma catecholamine assay. *Mayo Clinic Proceedings* **48**, 47.
Jones, N. F., Walker, G. *et al.* (1968). Alpha-methyl-paratyrosine in the management of phaeochromocytoma. *Lancet* **ii**, 1105.
Katz, R. L. and Wolf, C. E. (1971). Phaeochromocytoma. In *Highlights of Clinical Anesthesiology*. Ed. by L. C. Mark and S. H. Ngai. Harper and Row, New York and London.
Lawrence, C. A. (1978). Pethidine induced hypertension in phaeochromocytoma. *British Medical Journal* **1**, 149.
Leake, D., Carroll, J. J. *et al.* (1977). Management of phaeochromocytoma during pregnancy. *Canadian Medical Association Journal* **116**, 371.
Leather, H. M., Shaw, D. B. *et al.* (1962). Six cases of phaeochromocytoma with unusual clinical manifestations. *British Medical Journal* **1**, 1373.
Mason, G. A., Hart-Mercer, J. *et al.* (1957). Adrenaline-secreting neuroblastoma in an infant. *Lancet* **ii**, 322.
Mayo, C. H. (1927). Paroxysmal hypertension with tumor of retroperitoneal nerve. *Journal of the American Medical Association* **89**, 1047.
Melmon, K. L. (1968). The adrenals: part II: Catecholamines and the adrenal medulla. In: *Textbook of Endocrinology*, 4th edn, p. 379. Ed. by R. H. Williams. W. B. Saunders & Co., Philadelphia.
Murphy, M., Prior, F. N. *et al.* (1964). Halothane and blood transfusion for phaeochromocytoma: a case report. *British Journal of Anaesthesia* **36**, 813.
Nickerson, M. and Collier, D. (1975). Drugs inhibiting adrenergic nerves and structures innervated by them. In: *The Pharmacological Basis of Therapeutics*, 5th edn, p. 539. Ed. by L. S. Goodman and A. Gilman. Macmillan, New York.

Pincoffs, M. C. (1929). A case of paroxysmal hypertension associated with suprarenal tumor. *Transactions of the Association of American Physicians* **44**, 295.

Podolsky, S. and Pattavina, C. G. (1973). Hyperosmolar non ketotic diabetic coma, a complication of propranolol therapy. *Metabolism* **22**, 685.

Price, J. and Secher, O. (1961). Anaesthetic management of phaeochromocytoma. *Acta Anaesthesiologica Scandinavica* **5**, 153.

Richards, D. A. (1976). Pharmacological effects of labetalol in man. *British Journal of Pharmacology* **3**, Suppl. 3, 721.

Robertson, A. I. G. (1962). Anaesthetic management of phaeochromocytoma. *Proceedings of the Royal Society of Medicine* **54**, 432.

Robertson, A. I. G. (1965). Pre- and post-operative care of patients with phaeochromocytomas. *Postgraduate Medical Journal* **41**, 481.

Rollason, W. N. (1964). Halothane and phaeochromocytoma. *British Journal of Anaesthesia* **36**, 251.

Rosei, E. A., Brown, J. J. et al. (1976). Treatment of phaeochromocytoma and of clonidine withdrawal with labetalol. *British Journal of Pharmacology* Suppl., **3**, 809.

Ross, E. J., Pritchard, B. N. C. et al. (1967). Preoperative and operative management of patients with phaeochromocytoma. *British Medical Journal* **1**, 191.

Schnelle, N., Carney, F. M. T. et al. (1965). Anesthesia for surgical treatment of phaeochromocytoma. *Surgical Clinics of North America* **45**, 991.

Scott, D. B., Buckley, F. P. et al. (1976). Cardiovascular effects of labetalol during halothane anaesthesia. *British Journal of Pharmacology* Suppl., **3**, 817.

Seward, E. H. (1961). Death from phaeochromocytoma. *Lancet* **ii**, 903.

Sjoerdsma, A., Engelman, K. et al. (1966). Phaeochromocytoma. Current concepts of diagnosis and treatment. *Annals of Internal Medicine* **65**, 1302.

Smelley, J. M. and Sandler, M. (1961). Secreting intrathoracic ganglion neuroma. *Proceedings of the Royal Society of Medicine* **54**, 327.

Smith, A. M. (1973). Phaeochromocytoma and pregnancy. *Journal of Obstetrics and Gynaecology of the British Commonwealth* **80**, 848.

Stamenkovic, L. and Spierdijk, J. (1976). Anaesthesia in patients with phaeochromocytoma. *Anaesthesia* **31**, 941.

Swan, H. J. C. (1949). Effect of noradrenaline on the human circulation. *Lancet* **ii**, 508.

Szakacs, J. E. and Mehlman, B. (1960). Pathologic changes induced by L-norepinephrine. *American Journal of Cardiology* **5**, 619.

Van Way, C. W., Michelakis, A. M. et al. (1970). Renal vein renin studies in a patient with renal hilar phaeochromocytoma and renal artery stenosis. *Annals of Surgery* **172**, 212.

Van Way, C. W., Scott, H. W. et al. (1974). Pheochromocytoma. *Current Problems in Surgery* **2**, 59.

Van Way, C. W., Faraci, R. P. et al. (1976). Hemorrhagic necrosis of pheochromocytoma associated with phentolamine administration. *Annals of Surgery* **184**, 26.

Watkins, G. M., Johnson, T. D. *et al.* (1976). Phenoxybenzamine—a mediator of blood-oxygen affinity. *Journal of Trauma* **16,** 566.
Zintel, H. A., Eagle, J. F. *et al.* (1960). Phaeochromocytoma in children. *Surgery* **47,** 328.

Diabetes mellitus

Diabetes mellitus is a condition in which there is a reduction in insulin activity. It may be divided into primary and secondary diabetes. The primary condition may be further subdivided into juvenile or insulin-dependent, or adult type (which is non-insulin-dependent). The cause of primary diabetes is unknown but such factors as heredity, infection, stress, obesity and auto-immunity have been implicated (Cudworth, 1976).

The causes of secondary diabetes are listed below.

(1) Diabetes may be secondary to disorders of the pancreas such as pancreatitis and carcinoma.

(2) Growth hormone makes insulin less effective; diabetes is present in 30 per cent of patients with acromegaly.

(3) Excess secretion of adrenocortical hormones in Cushing's disease; where there is an increase in ACTH and adrenal glucocorticoids, there is a tendency to diabetes.

(4) Phaeochromocytoma. There is an increase in circulating pressor amines which antagonize the effects of insulin.

(5) Thyrotoxicosis; thyroid hormones increase the blood sugar by increasing the rate of absorption of glucose from the gut.

(6) In pregnancy there is often hyperglycaemia; there appears to be an increase in hormones which are antagonistic to the actual insulin.

(7) Drugs, such as thiazide derivatives (p. 105).

A deficiency in insulin leads to defects in the metabolism of carbohydrate, fat and protein. Thirst, polyuria, hyperglycaemia, glycosuria and ketonuria can occur with loss of water and electrolytes.

The function of insulin

Insulin has a molecular weight of about 6000 and is formed in the β cells of the pancreas from a precursor called proinsulin. Approximately 30–50 units of insulin are produced in the human per day; destruction is by the liver and elimination by the kidney.

Insulin promotes the entry of glucose into cells, where it is converted to glycogen. It inhibits lipolysis in adipose tissue, increases the potassium uptake by muscle and increases the uptake of amino acids into muscle protein. It inhibits the action of cyclic AMP.

In the absence of insulin, the following metabolic disorders will result: the blood sugar is raised due to less glucose entering into the cells. This results in hyperglycaemia and glycosuria; there is a decrease in glucose utilization and an increase in mobilization of fat into the blood stream, with an increase in concentration of triglyceride and free fatty acids (FFA); acetoacetic acid and β-hydroxybutyric acid are formed which result in metabolic acidosis; there is severe loss of sodium, potassium and water; protein is also broken down and the concentration of amino acids rises in the blood stream; large amounts of protein are converted to glucose.

Diagnosis

Patients may be symptomless and are only found to have diabetes on routine medical examination, when glycosuria is discovered. They may present with the symptoms of thirst, frequency of micturition, fatigue, loss of weight, pruritis and paraesthesia. They may also present as an acute fulminating case of diabetic coma precipitated by infection. The diagnosis may be made by testing the urine for sugar, performing a random blood sugar test when the level above 11 mmol/litre (200 mg/100 ml) will be highly suggestive, or by performing a glucose tolerance test.

Medical hazards associated with diabetes

(1) *Vascular disorders.* Arterial disease is common in diabetic patients, causing small vessel disease and poor peripheral pulses in the leg. Coronary artery disease is also more prevalent with an increased incidence of myocardial infarction.

(2) *Renal damage.* In the early stages there may be little renal damage, but with increasing damage of the capillaries in the glomeruli renal failure may occur.

(3) *The eye.* Cataract, retinal haemorrhages, microaneurysms, exudates and retinitis proliferans may be present.

(4) *Infection.* Diabetics are more prone to infection, particularly if they are poorly controlled. The urinary tract may be affected as well as the skin (e.g. carbuncle), and there may be an associated incidence of pulmonary tuberculosis. Infections are more likely to precipitate an attack of diabetic coma.

(5) *Neuropathy.* This may affect the autonomic, sensory and motor nerves.

(a) Autonomic. There may be disturbances of the bowel and bladder with postural hypotension, and an inability to respond to hypoglycaemia. Ewing *et al.* (1973) reported that the Valsalva manoeuvre was abnormal in 60 per cent of diabetic patients. Intermittent positive pressure ventilation (IPPV) could lead to a precipitous fall in blood pressure. Wheeler and Watkins (1973) noted cardiac denervation in diabetics, particularly of the vagus (Leading article, 1974). Postural hypotension has been provoked by insulin in diabetic neuropathies (Page and Watkins, 1976). Care should be taken with epidural analgesia. Page and Watkins (1978) also describe 12 cardiorespiratory arrests in 8 young diabetic patients with severe autonomic neuropathy. Five of these episodes occurred during or immediately after anaesthesia and were thought to be due to defective respiratory, rather than cardiovascular, reflexes. Pont *et al.* (1978) reported a similar case although they were unsure whether cardiac arrest had resulted from aspiration of gastric contents. Sanderson *et al.* (1978) suggest that young diabetics are particularly prone to suffer from cardiomyopathy.

(b) The sensory and motor nerves. The sensory and motor neuropathies may be acute or chronic, and patients may suffer from severe pain, paraesthesia, depressed tendon reflexes and loss of vibration sense; loss of sensation may lead to ulceration of the leg.

The neuromuscular junction may be defective in diabetic patients. In e.m.g. studies, the tetanus is poorly sustained, the action potential amplification decreased with stimulation of 50–100 Hz, even in muscles not clinically affected (Miglietta, 1973). The pathogenesis of diabetic polyneuropathy is discussed by Winegrad and Green (1976). The potential hazards of nerve block in patients with polyneuropathy should be considered in view of the possibility of an exacerbation of a neuropathy from local anaesthesic solutions, particularly those containing vasoconstrictors.

Treatment

The treatment of diabetes may be by:

(1) diet alone;
(2) diet and oral hypoglycaemic drugs;
(3) diet and insulin.

In the younger age group, there is evidence that the β cells are destroyed and therefore insulin will almost certainly be required. In the older age groups, the β cells still function but there is a delay in the initial response to insulin when glucose is given. Thus the mature diabetic may be controlled by diet, or by diet and oral hypoglycaemic drugs.

Insulin may be given in the soluble form, in which case the onset is rapid but the effect is short-lived. Long-acting insulins have a delayed onset and their release from tissue may depend on particle size (insulin zinc suspension) or the presence of zinc and protamine. The types of insulin are listed in Table 3.1.

Table 3.1   Insulin preparations in common use

Preparation	Maximum effect (hours)	Duration (hours)
Rapid and short-acting:		
Crystalline or soluble	2–4	6–8
Neutral (Actrapid MC)	1–3	5–7
Intermediate-acting:		
Isophane (NPH)	6–10	12–22
Biphasic (Rapitard)	1–3	20–24
	6–10	
Insulin zinc suspension, amorphous (semilente)	6–10	10–14
Delayed and long-acting:		
Protamine zinc insulin	12	36+
Insulin zinc suspension (lente) (mixture of 3 parts semilente and 7 parts ultralente)	6–10	20–24
Insulin zinc suspension, (ultralente)	12	36

Insulin

The advantage of isophane insulin is that it may be injected with soluble insulin while protamine insulin cannot be mixed with any other preparation. Rapitard (biphasic insulin BP) is a mixture of Actrapid (neutral insulin BP) and an intermediate acting ox insulin. Porcine insulin is said to be less antigenic than bovine insulin. There may be localized reactions to insulin, such as cutaneous allergy or atrophy of the subcutaneous fat at the site of injection (lipodystrophy). Generalized reactions may include anaphylactic reactions, arthritis and asthma.

More recently, insulins purified by anion chromatography have been introduced. These are devoid of proinsulin and are referred to as mono-component insulins. They are virtually non-antigenic and are 100 per cent porcine derived. In patients where insulin resistance is suspected, the mono-component insulin (MC) should be tried. Daily requirements of insulin will probably be less with MC insulin (Teuscher, 1975).

There are three mono-component insulins:

Neutral insulin (Actrapid).
Insulin zinc suspension (amorphous) (Semitard).
Insulin zinc suspension (Monotard).

There are three other insulins which contain less than 20 p.p.m. immunogenic proinsulin substances:

*Rapitard, which replaces the standard preparation of biphasic insulin.
*Lentard, Lente Novo, which replaces insulin zinc suspension.
*Ultratard, Ultralente Novo, which replaces insulin zinc suspension (crystalline).
(*These insulins are shortly to be replaced by equivalent MC insulins.)

Oral antidiabetic drugs

The oral antidiabetic drugs are only suitable for the mature diabetic who is producing insulin (Conley and Lowenstein, 1976; Alberti and Nattrass, 1977). They are divided into two groups: sulphonylureas and biguanides.

Sulphonylureas. These drugs stimulate the β cells of the pancreas to secrete insulin. They are well absorbed from the gastrointestinal tract and are effective by mouth. In general they are long-acting (Table 3.2) and are therefore

Table 3.2 Sulphonylureas

Preparation	Duration of action (hours)
Tolbutamide	8–12
Chlorpropramide	60
Glibenclamide	12–16

likely to cause hypoglycaemia. They can also cause blood dyscrasias, rashes, nausea and vomiting, and cholestatic jaundice. They should be used with care in patients with hepatic or renal disease. Facial flushing or headache may occur if alcohol is taken. The drugs are protein-bound and should be given with caution in patients who are having other drugs, such as sulphonamides, salicylates, phenylbutazone, anticoagulants and chloramphenicol. Amine oxidase inhibitors and propranolol are also contraindicated.

Biguanides. These drugs act not by releasing insulin from the pancreas but by increasing the peripheral utilization of glucose. Their side effects include anorexia, nausea and vomiting, and lactic acidosis. The drugs in common use are phenformin and metformin (Table 3.3).

It seems likely that phenformin will be restricted in its use to those patients under 60 years of age without cardiovascular or renal damage. When it is used, there should be frequent estimations of serum creatinine (Wise *et al.*, 1976).

Table 3.3.   Biguanides

Preparation	Duration of action (hours)
Phenformin	6–8
Metformin	5–6

Diabetes and surgery

Elective surgery

The management of patients undergoing surgery has become less hazardous in the last few years because of the ease with which it is possible to test urine for sugar and ketones, and the improved service which pathological laboratories are able to offer. Modern techniques of anaesthesia in general do not adversely affect diabetics although it must be remembered that these patients are prone to cardiovascular disorders and have impaired cardiovascular reflexes. Chloroform and ether are rarely used today; these drugs were widely implicated in adversely affecting diabetic patients by causing hyperglycaemia and possible liver damage.

In the preparation for surgery, no patient should be given oral glucose. Gastric emptying is delayed in diabetics (Scarpello *et al.*, 1976), while anxiety and preoperative sedation further delay absorption of the glucose solution (which is hypertonic). The use of oral glucose and insulin in preoperative preparation has no place in modern management, as during induction of anaesthesia glucose could readily be inhaled into the respiratory tract. The capricious absorption of the glucose may also lead to hypoglycaemia in the presence of the insulin. The commonest and most hazardous complication of surgery in diabetic patients is hypoglycaemia.

Patients without insulin. Patients treated by diet alone present little problem for their management at operation. Those on oral drugs should have the last dose on the day before operation, because the duration of action of chlorpropamide may be up to 60 hours. They may require insulin in the postoperative period, depending on the severity and duration of surgery.

Patients with insulin. For major surgery, patients should be admitted two to three days prior to surgery to assess and adjust the doses of insulin. Clarke and Duncan (1978) advocate that patients continue with long-acting insulin, the dose being adjusted so that the fasting blood glucose level is between 6·5 and 10 mmol/litre (117 and 180 mg/100 ml). If the level is between 6·5 and 14 mmol (117 and 252 mg), neither glucose nor insulin is given; if it is less than 6·5 mmol (117 mg) then an intravenous infusion of 5 per cent glucose is started and continued through operation. If it is above 14 mmol (252 mg), one-quarter to one-third of the usual daily dose of insulin is injected as NPH or IZS semilente. Thereafter, blood glucose determinations will determine the subsequent course of management as to whether more insulin is required.

At University College Hospital, London, it has been customary to change the patient's regimen to soluble insulin three times a day on the day prior to operation. On the day of operation, if it is to be performed in the morning, the following regimen is adopted. After induction of anaesthesia, half the normal dose of soluble insulin is given subcutaneously and intravenous infusion of 5 per cent dextrose started. For operations in the afternoon, the patient is given half the normal dose of insulin and a light breakfast; after induction of anaesthesia, half the normal dose of soluble insulin and an intravenous dextrose infusion is started. Thereafter the blood sugar and urine sugar are followed two- to four-hourly, and the doses of insulin and glucose to be given are based on these results.

These regimens impose a rigidity which is unnecessary and, at times, unhelpful. The rationale for the Clarke and Duncan regimen is based on the fact that—with the use of long-acting insulins—if hypoglycaemia were to occur, it would appear in the postoperative recovery period and would be readily recognized. The UCH regimen is based on the concept that the dose of soluble insulin is easier to adjust and that no insulin should be given without setting up an intravenous infusion. However, subcutaneous insulin may have an unreliable rate of absorption, especially in 'shock'.

Fletcher *et al.* (1965) made a study on 30 patients in the course of 36 operations. Blood sugar (preoperative) was measured when the premedication was given, and again when the patient was returned to the ward immediately following surgery (postoperative) (Fig. 3.14). No insulin or intravenous glucose was given during the course of surgery and there was very little disturbance of the blood sugar at operation; the mean change in the group was a rise of 0·39 mmol/litre (7 mg/100 ml). The study also showed that the dose of insulin (Fig. 3.15) and the type of insulin (Fig. 3.16) prior to surgery had little effect on the response of the blood sugar during surgery. Although the number of patients was small, it appeared that whether the operations were performed in the morning, mid-day or in the afternoon made little difference

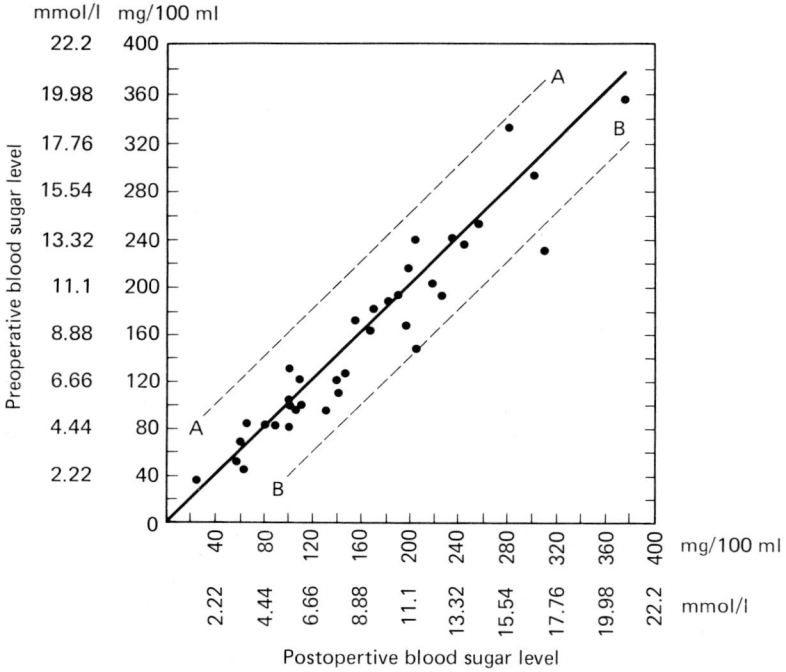

Fig. 3.14   Preoperative and postoperative blood sugar levels.

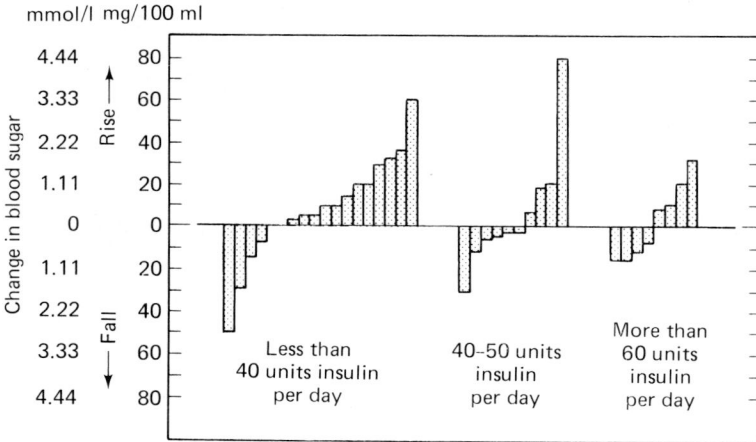

Fig. 3.15   Changes in blood sugar level, grouped according to the dose of insulin.

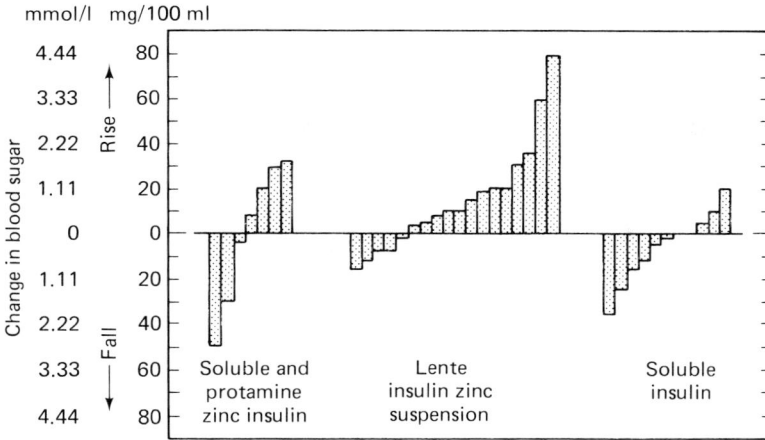

Fig. 3.16 Blood sugar levels, grouped according to the type of insulin.

to the effect on the blood sugar (Fig. 3.17). The severity of the operation did in fact cause a mean rise of 1·67 mmol/litre (30 mg/100 ml); this may be due to the fact that the duration of surgery was prolonged, and the blood sugar rose in the absence of insulin (Fig. 3.18).

There were 28 operations on patients whose diabetes was controlled by oral hypoglycaemic agents and there was a mean rise of only 0·78 mmol/litre (14 mg/100 ml) of blood sugar levels, but numbers in this group were small. However, when major operations occurred, the mean rise was 4·55 mmol/litre (82 mg/100 ml).

Thus it seems for major and intermediate surgery the arguments for insulin

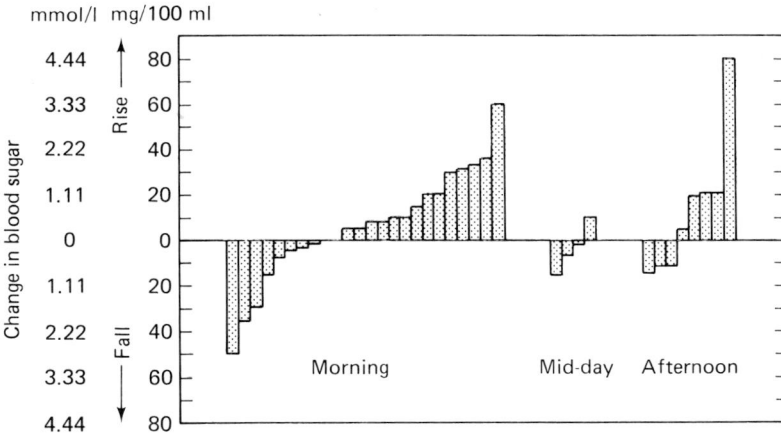

Fig. 3.17 Blood sugar levels, grouped according to the time of operation.

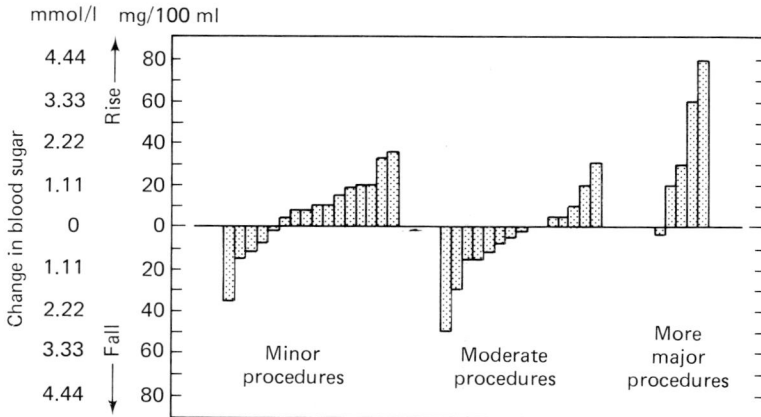

Fig. 3.18   Blood sugar levels, grouped according to the severity of operation.

and glucose regimens have been overstated, especially when blood sugar levels can readily be measured by an autoanalyser, or urine and blood sugars can be readily estimated by Clinitest and Dextrostix. Timing of the operation seems less critical than had formerly been supposed. However, scrupulous care is essential in the postoperative period, when possible nausea and vomiting which preclude the patient resuming his normal diet may necessitate the use of insulin and intravenous dextrose.

Major surgery. The following regimen is recommended, especially as it complies with the current concept of administering low doses of intravenous soluble insulin. For prolonged and extensive surgery, insulin can be added to the intravenous dextrose solution and administered at the rate of 2 units per hour. This has been shown to be more satisfactory than subcutaneous injections. The insulin is not readily destroyed in the solution (Clarke and Campbell, 1977). The dosage can be adjusted by following the blood sugar level. Three litres of intravenous dextrose 5 per cent or 4 per cent dextrose in 0·18 N saline per 24 hours and 2 units of insulin per hour form a useful baseline for management of major surgery. The dose of either can be varied according to the blood sugar estimation. Saline can be given to replace the dextrose solution. Hartmann's solution should not be used, as the lactate in 1 litre of solution can be converted to glucose by as much as 22 mmol/litre (396 mg/100 ml), increasing the plasma glucose concentration by 1–1·5 mmol/litre (18–27 mg/100 ml) (Thomas and Alberti, 1978). It is essential not to inject insulin into other solutions such as blood, or solutions containing antibiotics. The pH of soluble insulin is 3–3·5.

It must be remembered that during surgery under light anaesthesia there may be a hyperglycaemic response to stimulation. Insulin responses to glucose at operation have been studied by Giddings *et al.* (1977). Hypoglycaemia is readily recognized by sweating, tachycardia and dilated pupils. Griffiths (1953) showed, in both diabetics and non-diabetics, that the blood sugar fell if there was any hypotension. He also drew attention to the danger of ganglion-blocking drugs such as hexamethonium and of high spinal anaesthesia in producing a fall in blood sugar due to sympathetic blockade. The hypoglycaemia would be difficult to recognize in a diabetic on insulin, as the ganglion-blocking drug itself could produce tachycardia and dilated pupils, and interfere with sweating.

Emergency surgery. If the diabetes is severe and there is ketoacidosis it is advisable to control diabetes before surgery starts. (See management of diabetic coma, p. 100.) If the patient is in reasonable diabetic control then surgery may proceed, the blood sugar estimations determining thè amount of dextrose and insulin to be given. Possible electrolyte loss and dehydration should be considered in assessing further fluid loss at operation.

Minor operations. Minor elective surgical procedures present no major problems unless the patient has already had long-acting insulin on that day. The onset of hypoglycaemia is insidious, and recovery from operation may be delayed. It is advisable to admit patients to hospital for 24 hours under these circumstances.

Special precautions. Patients who are controlled by diet or oral hypoglycaemic agents may require insulin to be given for short periods after the operation. Patients on insulin will require a reduced dosage while in bed in hospital. Dextrostix estimations are unreliable at very low and very high levels of glucose. When there is a catheter *in situ*, urine specimens should be taken from the catheter itself and not from the drainage bag. During infection, the insulin requirements are increased, but when this is under control the dosage should be lowered correspondingly. In renal damage, the insulin requirements will be reduced. For operations on the mouth, as for tonsillectomy or removal of teeth, an intravenous infusion of saline should be set up during the course of surgery to ensure a vein is readily accessible for therapy. Patients may not take meals by mouth for 24–48 hours after these operations and it will be necessary to give insulin and dextrose intravenously as required.

Coma and hypoxaemia in diabetes

The causes of coma and hypoxaemia in diabetes are:

(1) diabetic ketoacidosis;
(2) hypoglycaemia;
(3) cerebral oedema;
(4) cerebral vascular accidents;
(5) disseminated intravascular coagulation;
(6) lactic acidosis;
(7) decreased red cell 2,3-diphosphoglycerate (2,3-DPG);
(8) hyperosmolar non-ketotic diabetic coma;
(9) drug interactions.

Diabetic ketoacidosis

This is due to insulin deficiency either as a result of the failure of the patient to receive his insulin, or due to increased requirements of insulin precipitated by stress (particularly infection) or because of the secretion of hormones which antagonize the action of insulin.

Symptoms. The patient may complain of thirst and have polyuria. There may be abdominal pain and vomiting. Weakness and drowsiness are present and there are signs of dehydration. A smell of acetone may appear in the patient's breath. Respiration may be sighing and eventually coma supervenes. Hyperventilation is well sustained with the metabolic acidosis except when acute tissue hypoxia exists (Fullop, 1976).

Mechanisms. Reduced insulin levels lead to hyperglycaemia and diminished glucose utilization. There is an increased mobilization of free fatty acids (FFA) which is accentuated by raised levels of hydrocortisone, growth hormone, glucagon and adrenaline. The FFA is converted in the liver to coenzyme A derivatives and oxidized to acetyl coenzyme A. Acetyl coenzyme A is normally handled by the acetic acid cycle, but in diabetes more is formed than can be destroyed. Acetyl coenzyme A is therefore converted to acetoacetic acid, β-hydroxybutyric acid and acetone. Although these ketone bodies are used for metabolic fuel, they accumulate in the blood stream. Protein breakdown is also increased. The increase in glucose and ketone bodies in the blood stream raises the osmolality over 330 mmol/kg (normal 283–300). Water leaves the cells and osmotic diuresis results with a loss of water which may exceed 6 litres. Sodium losses may amount to 500 mmol and potassium loss may exceed 400 mmol. Initially, the serum potassium may be normal or high due to tissue breakdown and this conceals the deficit. During treatment, potassium may drop markedly when potassium-free fluids are administered; potassium moves into the cells under the influence of insulin, and there is a continual loss by the kidney. The blood glucose level will be greater than 20 mmol/litre (360 mg/100 ml). There will be severe metabolic acidosis with a pH below 7·25. The P_{CO_2} will be reduced due to hyperventilation. Glucose is found in the urine, as are ketones. The serum bicarbonate may fall to 8 mmol/litre (8 mEq/litre) due to the ketonuria. Excess hydrogen ions also enter the cells, displacing potassium and further increasing the loss in the urine. Other electrolytes lost include: chloride; phosphate; magnesium, calcium and nitrogen due to tissue breakdown. Hyperventilation and vomiting increase fluid loss, leading to hypovolaemia and possible renal failure.

Treatment. Once the diagnosis has been established, treatment should be immediate. The management of diabetes essentially is to replace the fluid loss, the electrolyte loss, correct the acidosis, and administer insulin according to the arterial blood pH and blood gases, blood sugar, urea and electrolytes. Factors which have precipitated the attack of diabetic coma (such as infection) should be treated. The stomach should be aspirated and the patient carefully monitored, paying attention to pulse, blood pressure and respiration. The ECG should be monitored, especially to observe the effect of a possible low potassium. Oxygen should be administered if hypoxaemia is present. Catheterization of the patient should be avoided because of the risks of infection but may be necessary for fluid balance measurements.

As the expected fluid loss is about 6 litres and may be more, normal saline should be administered at the following rate:

First 2 hours	*First 6 hours*	*First 12 hours*
1·5–2 litres	3 litres	6 litres

Normal saline is given until the blood sugar is under 16·7 mmol/litre (300 mg/100 ml) and then 5 per cent glucose is substituted. If the serum sodium is greater than 155 mmol/litre (155 mEq/litre) then half normal saline should be given.

Insulin. Until recently it was fashionable to give insulin intravenously and intramuscularly in big doses—one recommendation was to give the dose in units approximately equivalent to twice the blood sugar level in millimoles or one-tenth of the blood sugar level in milligrams per 100 millilitres. However, the life of insulin is very short when given intravenously. Alberti *et al.* (1973) recommended the use of 10–20 units intramuscularly followed by hourly injections of 5–10 units. When the blood sugar falls below 13·9 mmol/litre (250 mg/100 ml) or when the urine sugar falls below 2 per cent, hourly injections of insulin are stopped and the patient is placed on a sliding scale of insulin on a six-hourly basis. Thus, for the sliding scale: 20 units should be given for 2 per cent glycosuria; 16 units for 1 per cent; 10 units for 0·5 per cent; 6 units for 0·25 per cent and zero for no glycosuria. This schedule has been modified by Page *et al.* (1974) and Kitson (1974), who advocate giving insulin intravenously by syringe pump or by a paediatric drip set at the rate of 8 units of soluble insulin per hour, thus delivering more physiological rates of insulin. This rate is continued until the ketosis is under control and the blood sugar is under 16·7 mmol/litre (300 mg/100 ml). The blood sugar under this regimen should fall at the rate of 4·2 mmol/litre (75 mg/ 100ml) per hour, when the infusion is stopped and insulin is given subcutaneously and intravenous dextrose administered. This method avoids hypoglycaemia, hypokalaemia and insulin resistance (Kitabchi *et al.*, 1976).

Semple *et al.* (1974) recommended that insulin be given at the rate of 0·1 unit/kg body weight per hour. The infusion solution is made by adding 50 units of insulin to 250 ml of saline and adding 3 ml of 25 per cent albumin to prevent adherence of the insulin to the plastic tubing (Kraegen *et al.*, 1975). Clarke and Campbell (1977) found the use of albumin unnecessary. When the blood glucose falls to 16·7 mmol/litre (300 mg/100 ml), intravenous glucose is substituted. When the blood glucose falls to 13·9 mmol/litre (250 mg/ 100 ml), this infusion may be discontinued if the ketones are no longer present and acidosis is corrected. If intravenous fluids are still required when the glucose level is 13·9 mmol/litre (250 mg/100 ml) the infusion rate of insulin is decreased to 0·02–0·05 units/kg body weight per hour, and 2–4 g glucose/ unit of insulin given to prevent hypoglycaemia. Clarke and Campbell (1977) showed that adults receiving an infusion of 6·5 units of insulin per hour had a fall in glucose of 5·5 mmol/litre (100 mg/100 ml) per hour, and the mean time in which serum ketones were cleared was six and one-half hours. The value of giving a continuous infusion is that the drug acts immediately. Subcutaneous injections absorb slowly and may last up to six hours, and in hypovolaemia the absorption is unpredictable. The plasma half-life of intravenous insulin is less than 5 minutes.

Potassium. Potassium is administered only if the urinary output is satisfactory, the blood sugar is falling and the serum potassium is under 5 mmol/litre (5 mEq). The requirements of potassium may be 20 mmol (20 mEq) in the first four hours, 50 mmol (50 mEq) in the first six hours and 90 mmol (90 mEq) in the first 12 hours. Potassium phosphate at the rate of 7–10 mmol per hour may be required.

Bicarbonate. Bicarbonate has been recommended if the arterial pH is less than 7 when approximately 100 mmol (100 mEq) (UCH preparation has 10 mmol of potassium and 5 mmol of phosphate in 10 ml) is given over half an hour. It has now become apparent that when insulin is given, ketones are metabolized via the Krebs cycle, and bicarbonate is regenerated. Another danger of giving bicarbonate is that a rise in blood pH may cause a decrease in CSF pH and a loss of consciousness. CO_2 crosses the blood–brain barrier quicker than bicarbonate. Intravenous bicarbonate causes a rise in blood pH but the hydrogen ion concentration falls and the stimulus for hyperventilation is lost. Increased CO_2 may cross the blood–brain barrier and cause a loss of consciousness (Kaye, 1975). However, these considerations must be set against the dangers of a pH of 7·1–7·2 when respiration is depressed and there are cardiac arrhythmias.

Osmolality. In the management of diabetes it is possible to measure serum osmolality but an approximation can be gained by the following formula:

Serum osmolality = 2 (Na ion + K ion) + glucose (mmol) + urea (mmol)

From this formula it can be seen that if the serum sodium ion concentration rises from 120 to 150 mmol/kg there will be an increase of 60 mmol/kg, a rise of blood glucose of 5·5 mmol/litre (100 mg/100 ml) adds approx. 5 mmol/litre and a rise of 1 mmol/litre (6 mg/100 ml) urea adds another 1 mmol/kg* (Chisholm, 1976).

Hypoglycaemia

Hypoglycaemia may occur during fasting (Ricketts, 1975; Fagans and Floyd, 1976). It has also been noted in children awaiting operation (Leading article,

---

* There is confusion between the terms osmolality and osmolarity. These have been freely interchanged, but strictly speaking osmolality is measured in mmol/kg and osmolarity is expressed in mmol per litre, and is no longer in current use; mmol/kg is the SI unit and mosm/kg is the conventional unit.

1976). However, in this context it usually results when antidiabetic drugs have been administered. Symptoms begin to develop when the blood sugar is at 2·8 mmol/litre (50 mg/100 ml), and is fully developed at 2·2 mmol/litre (40 mg/100 ml). In diabetics who have constantly high blood sugars, the level at which symptoms occur may be much higher.

Other causes of hypoglycaemia are islet cell tumour, ganglion-blocking drugs, high spinal epidural block and β-adrenergic-blocking agents. Hypoglycaemia is more common and comes on much more quickly than hyperglycaemic diabetic coma.

Diagnosis. The symptoms include weakness, sweating, palpitations, faintness, headaches and mental confusion. The symptoms are associated with increased production of adrenaline, resulting in tachycardia, tremor, sweating and dilated pupils.

Treatment. Treatment is by oral glucose, but if the patient is unable to swallow, 12·5 g of hypertonic glucose, 25 ml of 50 per cent solution, should be given intravenously.

Glucagon raises the blood sugar by mobilizing liver glycogen. Glucagon 1 mg intramuscularly raises the blood sugar but should be avoided in patients on long-acting insulin or those on oral antidiabetic drugs, as it stimulates insulin production. Glucagon is produced in the α cells of the pancreas, it acts by increasing adenyl cyclase which promotes the formation of cyclic AMP from adenosine triphosphate.

Diazoxide inhibits the secretion of insulin and has been used in the management of hypoglycaemia resulting from chlorpropamide (Johnson *et al.*, 1977).

Cerebral oedema

Cerebral oedema may occur from the over-rapid correction of increased osmolality. The inappropriate secretion of ADH has also been implicated.

Cerebral vascular accidents

Cerebral vascular accidents may occur due to hyperviscosity of the blood (Ditzel, 1977) and possible hypertensive or hypotensive episodes during operation.

Disseminated intravascular coagulation

Disseminated intravascular coagulation occurs not infrequently in diabetic ketoacidosis. Heparin therapy may be required, depending on the facilities for estimating platelets and fibrinogen degradation products (Nicholson and Tomkin, 1974).

Lactic acidosis

There are two main types of lactic acidosis: type A and type B. In type A, which is associated with clinical evidence of shock, there is clearly peripheral over-production of lactate and evidence of under-utilization. The prognosis is usually bad if acidosis is more than mild.

In type B lactic acidosis, there is no evidence of poor tissue perfusion and it occurs in patients taking phenformin (Woods, 1971; Cohen and Simpson, 1975). It also occurs in diabetic ketoacidosis, infections, hepatic disease, septicaemia, renal failure, acute alcoholism and in association with fructose infusion. The pH is less than 7·37 and blood lactate above 2 mmol/litre (18·02 mg/100 ml). The onset is rapid, hyperventilation is marked and consciousness may be lost. Hypotension and shock may develop later. Levels of 7 mmol/litre (63·07 mg/100 ml) of lactate are usually fatal. Treatment is with large amounts of sodium bicarbonate; up to 1000 mmol (1000 mEq) may be necessary in the first 36–48 hours. In the presence of an unexplained acidosis and an increased anionic gap, it is important to measure the blood lactate. The use of THAM and methylene blue has been advocated, as well as haemodialysis or peritoneal dialysis.

Decreased red cell 2,3-diphosphoglycerate (DPG)

The rapid correction of acidosis with bicarbonate may lead to disequilibrium in the pH between blood, brain and CSF. Bellingham *et al.* (1970) also drew attention to the problems associated with the rapid correction of metabolic acidosis in diabetes in relation to oxygen affinity for red cells. Using the term P50 which refers to the tension at which oxygen is 50 per cent saturated (26·6 mmHg, 3·5 kPa), they showed that when acidosis was induced there was an immediate decrease in oxygen affinity through the Bohr effect, but the decreased pH caused a delayed 2,3-DPG decrease which resulted in an increase in oxygen affinity. The lowered 2,3-DPG level balanced the effect of pH on the oxygen dissociation curve, so there is very little effect on the oxygen supply to tissues. Sudden correction of acidosis with bicarbonate caused an increase in the haemoglobin affinity for oxygen due to the Bohr effect. This effect is immediate whereas the correction of 2,3-DPG may take a few days to be complete (Alberti *et al.*, 1972; Ditzel, 1972, 1977).

Non-ketotic hyperosmolar diabetic coma (NKHC)

Non-ketotic hyperosmolar diabetic coma (NKHC) is a condition associated with dehydration, hyperglycaemia, hyperosmolality but no ketosis. The pathogenesis has been discussed by Joffe *et al.* (1975). The increase in free fatty acid levels which occurs during diabetic coma is blocked in NKHC so no ketones are formed. It has been reported to delay recovery from anaesthesia (Toker, 1974). The condition results from a shift of water to the intravascular space with intracellular dehydration. It is essentially an iatrogenic disease (Brenner *et al.*, 1973). It can arise in the following groups.

(1) Susceptible patients—those with diabetes, chronic pancreatitis, anaemia and those on cardiac bypass.
(2) Excessive glucose loads, as in giving dextrose, 50 per cent in hyperalimentation.
(3) Hyperglycaemic drugs—e.g. steroids, adrenaline.

(4) Dehydrating drugs, diuretics, thiazides.
(5) Uraemia.
(6) Extensive burns.
(7) Peritoneal dialysis.
(8) Drugs used for immunosuppression.
(9) Diazoxide and phenylhydantoin.
(10) Propranolol.

Treatment. The best form of treatment is prevention in this respect. In hyperosmolar coma without ketosis, the blood sugar may be as much as 66.6 mmol/litre (1200 mg/100 ml) and the serum osmolarity of 380 mmol/kg (380 mosm/kg). The patient should be rehydrated with isotonic saline followed by rapid infusion of 2–3 litres of hypotonic solution. If the serum sodium is high (as much as 150 mmol/litre) the hypotonic solution should be continued. Potassium is always needed; as much as 10–20 mmol (10–20 mEq) should be given every hour as well as 4–6 units of insulin intravenously per hour. Intravascular thrombosis is not uncommon.

Drugs in diabetes

Drugs given to diabetic patients may potentiate the actions of insulin or oral hypoglycaemic agents. Clonidine is now known to increase the action of insulin, resulting in hypoglycaemia. Adrenergic-blocking drugs such as propranolol are capable of producing NKHC (Podolsky and Pattavina, 1973) but are more likely to produce hypoglycaemia by enhancing the action of sulphonylureas and insulin. Metabolic responses to acute hypoglycaemia may be altered with β-adrenergic-blocking drugs (Decon *et al.*, 1977), especially acebutolol and propranolol. Salbutamol can induce ketoacidosis, while lithium may increase blood sugar (Johnson, 1977).

Drugs which are extensively protein-bound may displace other agents from plasma-protein-binding sites. This applies to phenylbutazone (98 per cent), warfarin (97 per cent) and tolbutamide (97 per cent). The action of tolbutamide is also intensified in the presence of sulphonamides.

Logie *et al.* (1976) discuss in detail the possible drug interactions, having found that control of diabetes on sulphonylureas was less effective in patients taking barbiturates or diuretics. Severe hypoglycaemia occurred in two patients taking phenylbutazone and chlorpropamide. They list the possible drug interactions in diabetic patients.

Diabetes in pregnancy

The management of pregnancy in diabetic patients has been dealt with in detail by Malins and Sulway (1972), and more recently by Essex (1976). In the regimen advocated by Essex, diabetics are managed by keeping the blood glucose levels below 8·3 mmol/litre (150 mg/100 ml). It is believed that if the maternal blood glucose level is high, fetal β cells produce insulin at 28 weeks. Excessive insulin results in excessive deposits of fat in the fetus. After delivery, the fetal insulin is still being produced, resulting in hypoglycaemia.

Insulin requirements rise by 50–100 per cent in the last three months of pregnancy. During labour the patient is given intravenous glucose and soluble insulin intravenously at a rate of 2–4 units per hour to keep the level of blood sugar between 3·66–5·55 mmol/litre (60 and 100 mg/100 ml). Labour is induced by rupturing the membranes; an oxytocin drip is commenced and the baby is carefully monitored with fetal scalp electrodes and repeated capillary blood samples where necessary. If the labour is not progressing satisfactorily after 8–10 hours, delivery is by caesarean section. Hypoglycaemia may develop in the mother, as the requirements of insulin drop dramatically within 1–2 hours of delivery. Hazards to the fetus include hypoglycaemia, polycythaemia, hyperbilirubinaemia, hypocalcaemia, and the respiratory distress syndrome (Roberts and Neff, 1976; Stubbs and Stubbs, 1978). Datta and Brown (1977) found that spinal anaesthesia for delivery resulted in a higher incidence of fetal acidosis in the diabetic: It was related to the degree of maternal diabetes and maternal hypotension following spinal anaesthesia.

References

Alberti, K. G. M. M. and Nattrass, M. (1977). Lactic acidosis. *Lancet* **ii,** 25.

Alberti, K. G. M. M., Darley, J. H. *et al.* (1972). 2,3-Diphosphoglycerate and tissue oxygenation in uncontrolled diabetes. *Lancet* **ii,** 391.

Alberti, K. G. M. M., Hockday, T. D. R. *et al.* (1973). Small doses of intramuscular insulin in the treatment of diabetic coma. *Lancet* **ii,** 515.

Bellingham, A. J., Datter, J. C. *et al.* (1970). The role of haemoglobin affinity for oxygen and red-cell 2,3-Diphosphoglycerate in the management of diabetic ketoacidosis. *Transactions of the Association of American Physicians* **83,** 113.

Brenner, W. I., Lenski, Z. *et al.* (1973). Hyperosmolar coma in surgical patients in iatrogenic disease of increasing incidence. *Annals of Surgery* **178,** 651.

Chisholm, D. J. (1976). Insulin therapy. *Medical Journal of Australia* **2,** 494.

Clarke, B. F. and Campbell, I. W. (1977). Direct addition of small doses of insulin to intravenous infusion in severe uncontrolled diabetes. *British Medical Journal* **2,** 1395.

Clarke, B. F. and Duncan, L. J. P. (1978). Diabetes mellitus. In: *Textbook of Medical Treatment*, 14th edn, p. 269. Ed. by S. Alstead and R. H. Girdwood. Churchill Livingstone, London and New York.

Cohen, R. D. and Simpson, R. (1975). Lactate metabolism. *Anesthesiology* **43,** 661.

Conley, L. A. and Lowenstein, J. E. (1976). Phenformin and lactic acidosis. *Journal of the American Medical Association* **235,** 1575.

Cudworth, A. G. (1976). The aetiology of diabetes mellitus. *British Journal of Hospital Medicine* **16,** 207.

Datta, S. and Brown, W. U. (1977). Acid base status in diabetic mothers and their infants following general or spinal anesthesia for cesarian section. *Anesthesiology* **47,** 272.

Decon, S. B., Karunanayake, A. *et al.* (1977). Acebutolol, atenolol and propranolol and metabolic responses to acute hypoglycaemia in diabetics. *British Medical Journal* **2,** 1255.

Ditzel, J. (1972). Impaired oxygen release caused by alterations of metabolism in diabetes. *Lancet* **i,** 721.

Ditzel, J. (1977). Increased oxygen affinity and blood viscosity in diabetes. *Lancet* **ii,** 184.

Essex, N. (1976). Diabetes in pregnancy. *British Journal of Hospital Medicine* **15,** 333.

Ewing, D. J., Campbell, I. W. *et al.* (1973). Vascular reflexes in diabetic autonomic neuropathy. *Lancet* **ii,** 1354.

Fagans, S. S. and Floyd, J. C. (1976). Fasting hypoglycemia in adults. *New England Journal of Medicine* **294,** 766.

Fletcher, J., Langman, M. J. S. *et al.* (1965). Effect of surgery on blood sugar levels in diabetes mellitus. *Lancet* **ii,** 52.

Fullop, M. (1976). The ventilatory response of severe metabolic acidosis. *Clinical Science and Molecular Medicine* **50,** 367.

Giddings, A. E. B., Mangnali, D. *et al.* (1977). Plasma insulin and surgery. 1. Early changes due to operation in insulin response to glucose. *Annals of Surgery* **186,** 681.

Griffiths, J. A. (1953). Effects of general anaesthetics and hexamethonium on blood sugar. *Quarterly Journal of Medicine* **22,** 405.

Joffe, B. I., Goldberg, R. B. *et al.* (1975). Pathogenesis of nonketotic hyperosmolar diabetic coma. *Lancet* **i,** 1069.

Johnson, B. B. (1977). Diabetes mellitus in patients on lithium. *Lancet* **ii,** 935.

Johnson, S. F., Schade, D. S. *et al.* (1977). Chlorpropamide induced hypoglycemia. Successful treatment with diazoxides. *American Journal of Medicine* **63,** 799.

Kaye, R. (1975). Diabetic ketoacidosis—the bicarbonate controversy. *Journal of Pediatrics* **87,** 156.

Kitabchi, A. E., Ayyagar, I. V. *et al.* (1976). The efficacy of low dose *v.* conventional therapy of insulin for treatment of diabetic ketoacidosis. *Annals of Internal Medicine* **84,** 633.

Kitson, W., Casey, J. *et al.* (1974). Treatment of severe diabetes mellitus by insulin infusion. *British Medical Journal* **2,** 691.

Kraegen, E. W., Lazarus, L. *et al.* (1975). Carrier solutions for low-level intravenous insulin infusion. *British Medical Journal* **3,** 464.

Leading article (1974). Diabetic autonomic neuropathy. *British Medical Journal* **3,** 2.

Leading article (1976). Hypoglycaemia in children undergoing adeno-tonsillectomy. *British Medical Journal* **1,** 751.

Logie, A. W., Galloway, D. B. *et al.* (1976). Drug interactions and long-term antidiabetic therapy. *British Journal of Clinical Pharmacology* **3,** 1027.

Malins, J. M. and Sulway, M. J. (1972). Management of diabetes in pregnancy, surgery and inter-current illness. *British Journal of Hospital Medicine* **17,** 201.

Miglietta, O. (1973). Neuromuscular junction defect in diabetes. *Diabetes* **22**, 719.

Nicholson, G. and Tomkin, G. H. (1974). Successful treatment of disseminated intravascular coagulopathy complicating diabetic coma. *British Medical Journal* **4**, 450.

Page, M. M., Alberti, K. G. M. M. *et al.* (1974). Treatment of diabetic coma with continuous low dose infusion of insulin. *British Medical Journal* **2**, 687.

Page, M. M. and Watkins, B. J. (1976). Provocation of postural hypotension by insulin in diabetic autonomic neuropathy. *Diabetes* **25**, 90.

Page, M. M. B. and Watkins, B. J. (1978). Cardio-respiratory arrest and diabetic autonomic neuropathy. *Lancet* **i**, 14.

Podolsky, S. and Pattavina, C. G. (1973). Hyperosmolar non-ketotic diabetic coma, a complication of propranolol therapy. *Metabolism* **22**, 685.

Pont, A., Rushing, J. L. *et al.* (1978). Cardiorespiratory arrest in diabetic neuropathy. *Lancet* **i**, 386.

Ricketts, H. T. (1975). Hypoglycaemia during fasting. *Journal of the American Medical Association* **234**, 186.

Roberts, M. F. and Neff, R. K. (1976). Maternal diabetes and the respiratory distress syndrome. *New England Journal of Medicine* **294**, 357.

Sanderson, J. E., Brown, D. J. *et al.* (1978). Diabetic cardiomyopathy? An echocardiographic study of young diabetics. *British Medical Journal* **1**, 404.

Scarpello, J. H. B., Barber, D. C. *et al.* (1976). Gastric emptying solid meals in diabetics. *British Medical Journal* **2**, 671.

Semple, E., White, C. *et al.* (1974). Continuous infusion of small doses of insulin in the treatment of diabetic ketoacidosis. *British Medical Journal* **2**, 694.

Stubbs, W. A. and Stubbs, S. M. (1978). Hyperinsulinism, diabetes mellitus, and respiratory distress of the newborn: a common link? *Lancet* **i**, 308.

Teuscher, A. (1975). The place of mono-components in the therapy of diabetes mellitus. *Schweizerische Medizinische Wochenschrift* **105**, 485.

Thomas, D. J. B. and Alberti, K. G. M. M. (1978). Hyperglycaemic effect of Hartmann's solution during surgery in patients with maturity onset diabetes. *British Journal of Anaesthesia* **50**, 185.

Toker, E. R. (1974). Hyperosmolar, hyperglycaemic non-ketotic coma, a cause of delay in recovery from anaesthesia. *Anaesthesia* **41**, 284.

Wheeler, T. and Watkins, B. J. (1973). Cardiac denervation in diabetes. *British Medical Journal* **4**, 584.

Winegrad, A. I. and Green, D. A. (1976). Diabetic polyneuropathy. The importance of insulin deficiency, hyperglycemia and alterations in myoinositol metabolism in its pathogenesis. *New England Journal of Medicine* **295**, 1416.

Wise, P. H., Chapman, M. *et al.* (1976). Phenformin and lactic acidosis. *British Medical Journal* **1**, 70.

Woods, H. F. (1971). Some aspects of lactic acidosis. *British Journal of Medicine* **7**, 868.

Thyroid

The thyroid gland was first described in the seventeenth century, and the fluid within it was thought to be necessary to lubricate the trachea. It was in the late nineteenth century that its importance was realized, especially its effect on metabolic rate.

The active principles of the thyroid glands are synthesized in the follicular cells and are thyroxine (T_4) and tri-iodothyronine (T_3). Thyroxine was isolated in crystalline form in 1915 but it was not until 1952 that T_3 was finally synthesized. T_3 is ten times less bound to plasma protein (globulin) than T_4, hence T_3 acts more quickly on tissues and has a shorter half-life. Between the follicles of the thyroid gland are parafollicular cells (C cells) and it was only in 1961 that it was realized that these were responsible for the production of calcitonin (p. 118).

Synthesis of thyroid hormones

Iodine is an essential constituent of the thyroid hormones and is ingested in the form of iodide. It is concentrated in the colloid of the thyroid gland and converted by peroxidases to iodine. The iodine is taken up by tyrosine to form monoiodotyrosine and diiodotyrosine. These compounds unite to form thyroxine and tri-iodothyronine. T_3 and T_4 are synthesized and stored as part of the molecule of thyroglobulin in the colloid vesicles.

The anterior pituitary gland secretes thyroid-stimulating hormone, thyrotrophin (TSH), which promotes the release of thyroid hormones from the colloid and also stimulates the synthesis of the thyroid hormones. There is increased vascularity of the gland. It is possible that thyrotrophin (TSH) may activate the thyroid by promoting an increase in adenyl cyclase and thereby increase the concentration of cyclic AMP. There is a negative feedback mechanism in that the thyroid hormones can inhibit secretion of thyrotrophin. TSH secretion is also under the control of the hypothalamus (thyrotrophin-releasing hormone; TRH).

Metabolism of thyroid hormones

In normal persons, thyroxine has a half-life of six or seven days. In hyperthyroidism the half-life is shortened, but in myxoedema it is prolonged. The globulin which binds thyroxine is increased in pregnancy and therefore the elimination of thyroxine is delayed. In cirrhosis of the liver the converse applies and elimination is increased. Thyroxine is degraded in the liver and conjugated with glucuronic acid.

Action of thyroid hormones

Thyroxine stimulates metabolism in tissues, increasing oxygen consumption and heat production. There are increases in metabolic rate, cardiac output, heart rate and cardiac work. Thyroxine is necessary for growth and development of most tissues but in excess it causes tissue breakdown, especially of protein. It promotes the absorption of glucose, raises the blood sugar and reduces serum cholesterol. It causes diuresis with loss of potassium. The effects are more obvious in conditions of over- and under-secretion (see below and pp. 116, 117).

Thyroid function tests

Tests of thyroid function have been reviewed by McConnon (1973) and Harvard (1974a). These include the measurement of (1) ^{131}iodine uptake; (2) T_3 suppression; (3) T_3 resin uptake; (4) protein-bound iodine; (5) total serum thyroxine (T_4); (6) TSH in response to TRH released by the hypothalamus; and (7) thyroid antibody.

Goitre

The enlargement of the thyroid gland may be due to: (1) simple colloid goitre from iodine deficiency; (2) lymphadenoid goitre, Hashimoto's thyroiditis; (3) Riedel's goitre; (4) carcinoma; and (5) thyroiditis. Goitre may occur in association with thyrotoxicosis.

Simple goitre

This is due to the deficiency of iodine. There is an increase in TSH, causing increase in the size of the gland. Treatment is with potassium iodide 60 mg per day to correct the iodine deficiency, and with thyroid in the form of synthetic L-thyroxine 0·1–0·3 mg per day, to inhibit TSH production. In Hashimoto's thyroiditis, when antibodies to thyroglobulin are often present, goitre and hypothyroidism may coexist. Thyroxine should be given 0·2–0·3 mg per day and continued indefinitely. Carcinoma of the thyroid is usually treated by excision, palliative radiotherapy and the administration of thyroxine.

Hyperthyroidism

This is associated with the over-production of T_3 and of T_4. The blood levels of TSH are not increased, but there is an abnormal γ-globulin called long-acting thyroid stimulator (LATS), which is increased.

Symptoms

Symptoms are those of increased metabolism with increase in cardiac output, tachycardia and arrhythmias; signs of cardiac failure are more likely to occur in the elderly. There are signs of increased sympathetic activity, excitability, diarrhoea and tremor, while the hands are hot and sweaty. Other features include loss of weight, increased tendon reflexes, proximal weakness (myopathy), retraction of the upper eyelids and exophthalmos which is believed to be due to LATS secretion. The blood sugar may be raised and there is a reduction in plasma cholesterol. The thyroid may be enlarged.   ·

Treatment of thyrotoxicosis

Thyrotoxicosis is treated with antithyroid drugs, radioactive iodine or by surgery. The β-adrenergic-blocking drugs also have a place in the management of hyperthyroidism (Harvard, 1974b).

Antithyroid drugs

Thionamides. Antithyroid drugs act by interfering with the uptake of iodine into an organic form. The drug commonly used in the UK is carbimazole; it is given in the dose of 10–15 mg every 6 hours for one to two weeks. After this period, the dose can be adjusted to a maintenance level of the order of 10–15 mg per day. In other centres (Evered, 1976) the full blocking dose of carbimazole is maintained and 0·15 mg thyroxine given daily as well.

Adverse reactions to antithyroid drugs include agranulocytosis, urticaria, jaundice and drug fever. Alternative antithyroid drugs may be prescribed, such as methylthiouracil or propylthiouracil in the initial dose of 300–400 mg per day and a maintenance dose of 100 mg per day.

Potassium perchlorate, which interferes with iodine transport, should be used only in those who develop a dyscrasia to thionamides.

Radioactive iodine

This is suitable for patients over the age of 40 who develop thyrotoxicosis, and for those who have had attacks of cardiovascular failure. They may require control of their cardiovascular system with digoxin and diuretics and may also need carbimazole.

Surgery

Surgical treatment is indicated in the young thyrotoxic patient with a large goitre and in those in whom medical treatment has been unsuccessful.

Preparation of the patient for surgery

Hyperthyroid patients are prepared for thyroidectomy with carbimazole 10 mg t.d.s. for three to six weeks. Propranolol 40 mg q.i.d. is of value in antagonizing any sympathetic over-activity; however, this drug must be avoided in patients with cardiac failure or asthma. The vascularity of the thyroid gland can be decreased by the administration of potassium iodide 60 mg t.d.s. for ten days preoperatively. McDevitt (1977) comments that this long preparation for surgery is unnecessary, and that propranolol 40–180 mg 6-hourly for four days gives adequate preparation of the patient for surgery remembering that the patients are still hyperthyroid and will require treatment with β blockers for seven to ten days postoperatively. While awaiting surgery patients should be adequately sedated with phenobarbitone 30–60 mg per day, or with diazepam 5 mg t.d.s. In addition to the investigations for thyroid activity, it is important whenever operating on a thyroid gland that adequate

(a)

(b)

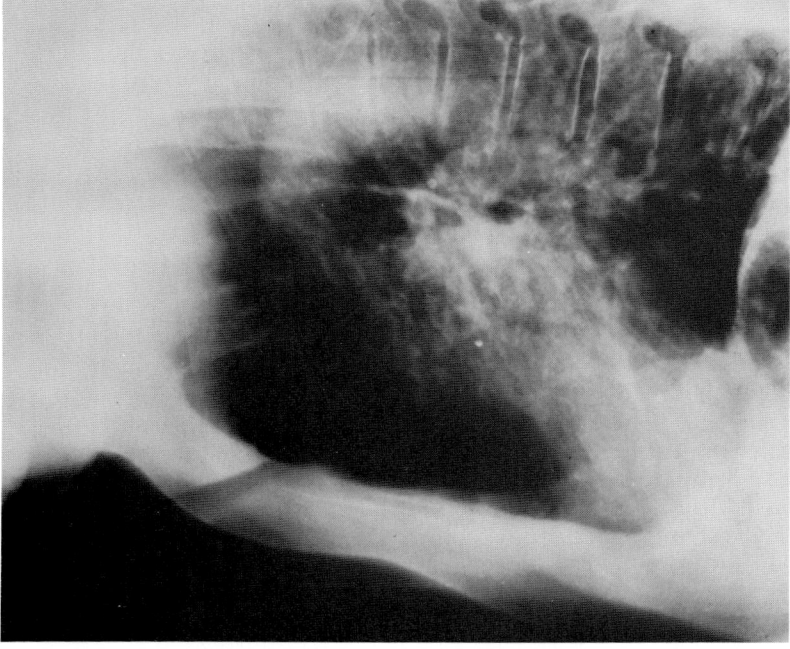

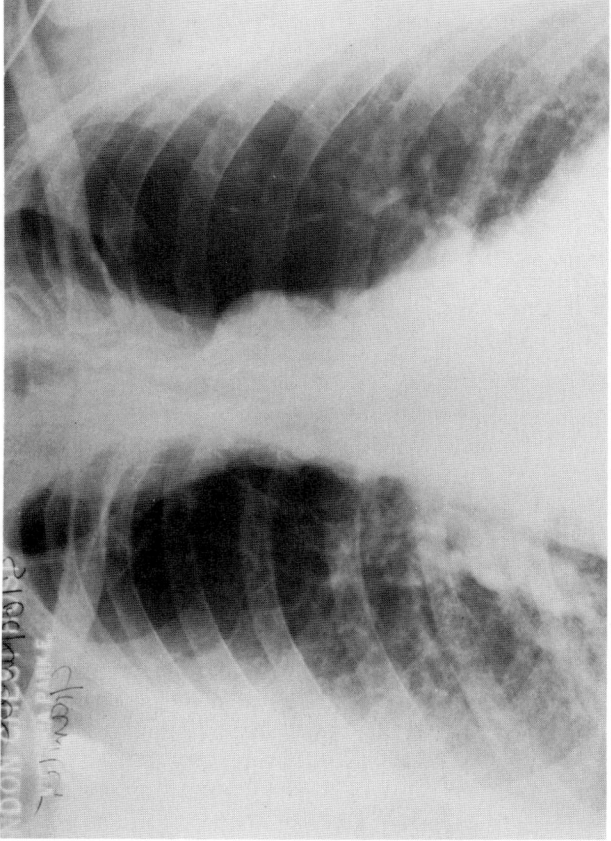

Fig. 3.19 (a and b) Retrosternal goitre, showing compression of trachea.

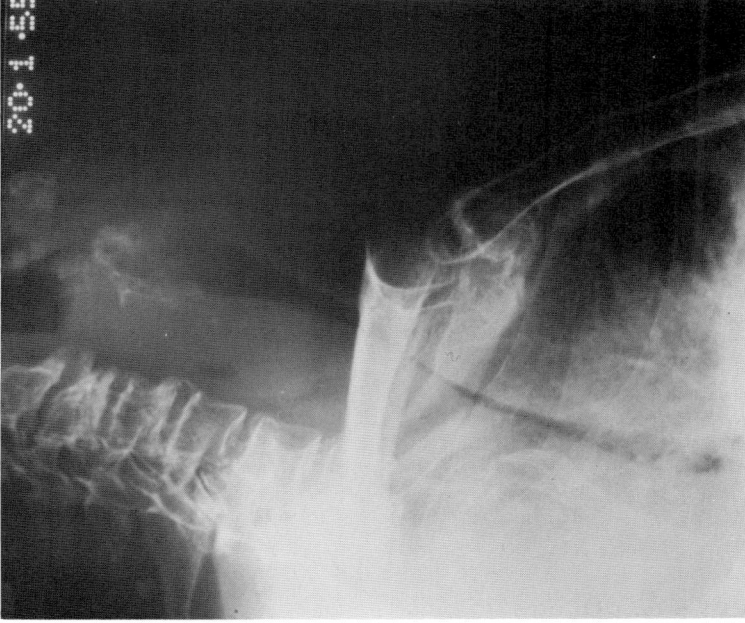

(b)

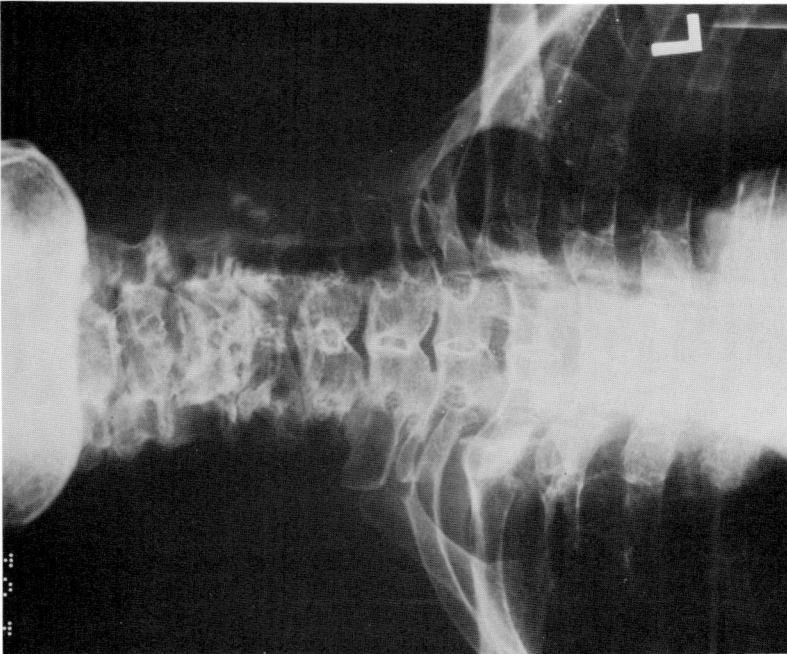

(a)

Fig. 3.20 (a and b) Carcinoma of the thyroid, showing displacement to the left and narrowing of the trachea.

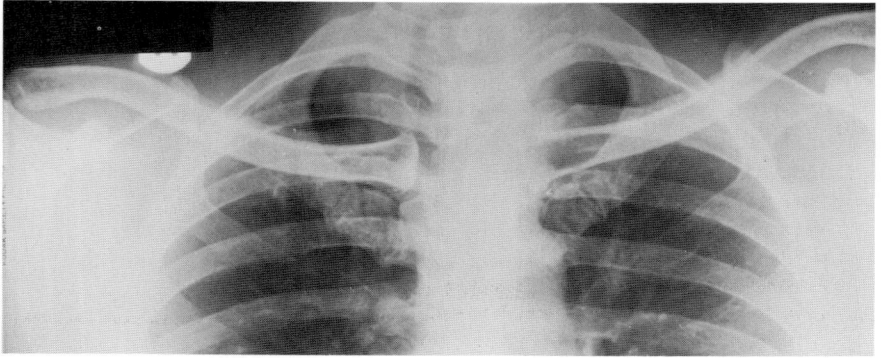

(a)

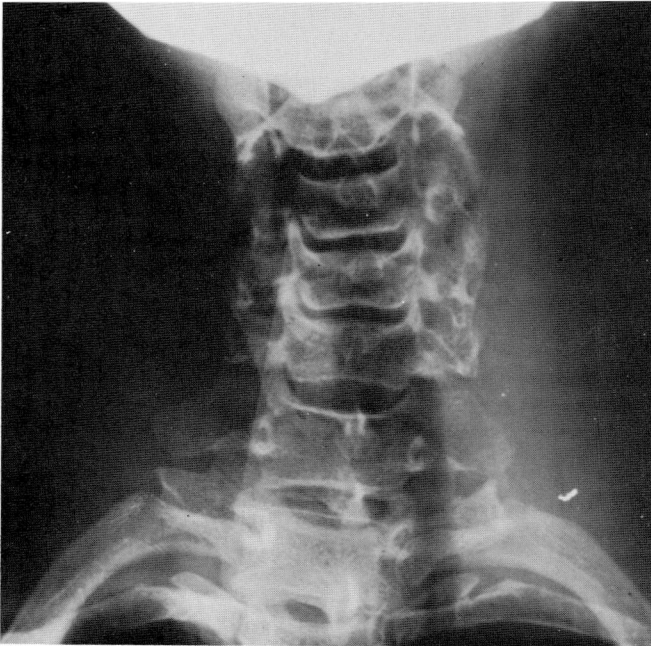

(b)

Fig. 3.21   (a and b) Goitre, causing deviation to the right of the trachea.

x-rays should be taken to determine whether there is compression or deviation of the trachea or any retrosternal prolongation of the thyroid gland (Figs. 3.19–3.21).

Anaesthetic management

Adequate premedication should ensure that the patient comes to the operating theatre in a relaxed state. The historic practice of 'stealing the thyroid' consisted of preparing the patient daily with enemas but, on the day of operation, the bland fluid was replaced either by tribromoethyl alcohol (Bromethol) or paraldehyde. The good intentions of this technique were easily thwarted by patients informing those awaiting surgery of the particular day on which the surgeon customarily operated. Premedication may consist of diazepam, or papaveretum and hyoscine. Atropine should be avoided because of its effects on cardiac rate and cardiac output, and it can inhibit sweating. As the metabolic rate is raised, drugs will be destroyed more rapidly than usual.

General anaesthetic techniques include an intravenous barbiturate, a short-acting relaxant for intubation, applying lignocaine spray to the vocal cords, the atraumatic passage of a non-kinkable and non-compressible endotracheal tube. Anaesthesia can be maintained by any appropriate technique. Nitrous oxide, oxygen and halogen, with or without paralysis and artificial ventilation, may be used. Alternatively, intermittent injections of analgesics such as pethidine or fentanyl may be preferred to halothane. By carefully posturing the patient with a slight head-up tilt, venous oozing may be reduced. The eyes, particularly if there is exophthalmos, should be carefully protected. The surgeon may wish to infiltrate the line of incision and the soft tissues with saline or adrenaline (not more than 50 ml of 1 : 200 000 injected slowly, care being taken to avoid inadvertent intravenous injection). The latter is not contraindicated in the presence of halothane provided the P_{CO_2} is not elevated, the patient is not toxic and the pulse rate is carefully monitored. Prior administration of β blockers may prevent ventricular ectopic beats, which can also be controlled at operation with propranolol 0·5–1 mg intravenously. The use of hyoscine for premedication can result in bradycardia (central effect) which may further slow the heart rate in the presence of propranolol.

Local anaesthetic techniques are rarely performed today for thyroidectomy.

Complications of operation

These may be divided into:

    (1) Immediate:
        (a) respiratory obstruction;
        (b) hyperthyroid crisis;
        (c) tetany;
        (d) eye complications.
    (2) Late—hypothyroidism.

Respiratory obstruction. (1) Haemorrhage. Respiratory obstruction may result from haemorrhage which can compress the trachea; treatment involves the emergency removal of stitches and evacuating the haematoma.

(2) Trauma. The larynx may become oedematous as a result of traumatic intubation associated with infection and from the external trauma of surgery. Presterilized endotracheal tubes obviate many of the former problems and using the recently introduced siliconed endotracheal tubes reduces the trauma to the mucosa of the larynx and trachea.

(3) Tracheal collapse. This has been mentioned as a cause of respiratory obstruction. It was believed that the rings of trachea were softened by the pressure on the larynx.

(4) Nerve damage. Respiratory obstruction may result from damage of either or both the recurrent laryngeal nerves during dissection in the neck. Inspection of the vocal cords at the end of the operation is not always a reliable guide as to the integrity of these nerves. Should recurrent nerve damage be apparent in the immediate postoperative period, immediate reintubation is advised. A hoarse or croaking voice after the operation may be caused by damage to the external laryngeal branch of the superior laryngeal nerve; this supplies cricoid thyroid muscle which tenses the vocal cord.

Hyperthyroid crisis. This is due to the sudden increase in thyroid activity seen after surgery in those patients who have been inadequately prepared. The patient may become delirious, suffer severe mental and physical exhaustion, and become dehydrated, ketotic and comatose. High temperature with tachycardia is often present and cardiac failure may ensue. The standard treatment of thyrotoxic crisis has been to give potassium iodide 300–6000 mg i.v., to administer intravenous fluid to combat the dehydration and to treat the hyperpyrexia with chlorpromazine. Antithyroid drugs, such as carbimazole, were started as soon as the patient was able to tolerate them orally. Hydrocortisone 100–300 mg could be given intravenously to combat the relative steroid insufficiency. Temperature could also be controlled by aspirin, tepid sponging or the application of ice packs to the limbs. Oxygen was also administered. Digoxin and diuretics were given to combat cardiac failure. However, the treatment of choice now consists of giving propranolol 1 mg per minute intravenously, to a maximum of 5 mg, taking great care to monitor the blood pressure.

Tetany. This may occur in the postoperative period by removal or a temporary interruption of the blood supply of the parathyroid glands. The blood calcium or the ionized form is reduced as a result, and treatment consists of 10 per cent calcium gluconate intravenously 20 ml over a period of 5 minutes. For more prolonged therapy, calciferol 1·25 mg t.d.s. should be given, but the serum calcium concentration should be monitored to avoid the blood level exceeding 2·62 mmol/litre (10·5 mg/100 ml). As an alternative dihydrotachysterol (AT 10) can be given.

Eye complications. In thyrotoxicosis there may be lid retraction exophthalmos and ophthalmoplegia. Exophthalmos can be complicated by conjunctivitis, diplopia and oedema of the conjunctiva. Treatment is not entirely satisfactory, but discomfort in the eye may be treated with methylcellulose eye-drops. Guanethidine eye-drops may be of value, but unfortunately they often irritate the conjunctiva.

At operation the eyes, which may be prominent because of exophthalmos, may be damaged by pressure from assistants resulting in corneal abrasions. The eyes should be carefully closed, sealed with adhesive tape and padded.

Hypothyroidism. This may be a late complication of thyroid surgery. It may be due to thyroid deficiency at birth, in which case cretinism develops, or it may arise later in life after normal physical development has taken place, resulting in juvenile hypothyroidism. The latter is readily treatable if diagnosed early.

In the adult, hypothyroidism may occur from primary thyroid failure, decreased thyrotrophic hormone from the pituitary or the hypothalamus or from circulating antibodies as seen in Hashimoto's thyroiditis. Oral treatment with antithyroid drugs is another cause and this includes not only carbimazole but also radioactive iodine.

The patients are sensitive to cold, are easily tired, have a poor appetite and lose weight. The skin is dry, the eyelids may be puffy, the lips thickened and the tongue enlarged. The skin may be thickened, giving the characteristic appearance of myxoedema. Speech may be slow. The metabolic rate is lowered; there may be hypothermia, hypoglycaemia and depressed reflexes. The heart is often enlarged and the pulse may be slow. The serum cholesterol is raised, predisposing to atheroma. The patients may develop psychosis, coma and hypothermia.

The major features of interest to anaesthesia are that the reduced metabolic rate implies that drugs will be metabolized at a very much slower rate. Furthermore, with hypothermia, drug action may also be prolonged.

The test of choice to confirm hypothyroidism is the protein-bound iodine.

Treatment consists of oral thyroxine 0·1 mg per day, increasing to 0·2 mg after a month. Rapid increase in the dose may result in angina or cardiac failure. It may be necessary to use propranolol to control the angina in patients being treated with thyroxine.

In patients with myxoedematous coma T_3 5–10 μg may be given intravenously; hydrocortisone should also be given and the body temperature raised slowly. Assisted ventilation may be required, as may intravenous fluids. Careful monitoring of blood pressure and blood gases is often necessary.

Parathyroid

Parathyroid hormone (PTH) is formed in the parathyroid glands from a prohormone. It consists of 84 amino acids and has a molecular weight of about 10 000. Its main function is to maintain the concentration of calcium in cellular and extracellular fluids. Secretion of PTH is determined by the concentration of ionized calcium in the blood: a fall in serum calcium results in increased secretion of PTH whereas a rise in serum calcium depresses the level of PTH secretion. PTH acts on kidney and bone; it may do this by acting on the intracellular cyclic AMP (Tomlinson and O'Riorden, 1978). PTH increases the absorption of calcium from the intestine and the mobilization of calcium phosphate in bone, and decreases the excretion of calcium. Its effects on intestine and bone require vitamin D. It increases the excretion of phosphate. As the plasma levels of calcium rise there is an increased filtration of calcium and excretion in the urine.

Calcitonin, which is secreted by the thyroid gland, antagonizes the action of parathormone. Its main effect is to lower the serum calcium by transferring it to bone. Phosphate levels are also lowered.

Primary hyperparathyroidism

Renal colic—due to calcium stones—is common as well as gastrointestinal disturbances. There is often weight loss, with dyspepsia, anorexia and generalized aches and pains. Dyspnoea, hypotension, cardiac arrhythmias and polyuria can occur and, in the acute state, dehydration may ensue (Tomlinson and O'Riorden, 1978). Acute pancreatitis is sometimes a feature. Cysts may appear on the bone.

There is an increase in the plasma concentration of calcium, which may reach 5 mmol/litre (20 mg/100 ml); (normal 2·25–2·55 mmol/litre; 9–10·2 mEq/100 ml). Estimation of ionized calcium is more difficult than that of total calcium. Half the calcium is protein bound to albumin, and allowances must be made for variations in plasma albumin. The tests include measurements of calcium and phosphate levels in the urine, the hydrocortisone suppression test and the assay of PTH.

Treatment. The treatment of acute hypercalcaemia consists of correcting dehydration with intravenous fluids. Intravenous phosphate, sodium sulphate, EDTA, steroids and calcitonin have been used to reduce the serum calcium. Haemodialysis may be required.

The surgical removal of the parathyroid glands may be technically difficult because they may extend into the mediastinum. Management of patients for operation may be influenced by the fact that there may be renal damage, in which case there may be hazards associated with excretion of drugs. In addition, because there is osteoporosis and generalized weakness, respiratory function may be impaired and there is danger in causing fracture of bones in moving patients (Figs. 3.22–3.24, see pp. 119, 120). After parathyroidectomy the plasma Ca falls to normal within 48 hours, but if it continues to fall tetany may result because reduction in calcium ions leads to membrane instability resulting in spontaneous action potentials. Calcium is also necessary for release of ADH, catecholamines and acetylcholine at the neuromuscular junction.

Hypoparathyroidism

Hypoparathyroidism may occur after the removal of the thyroid gland. It may be transitory due to interference with the blood supply to the parathyroid or it may be permanent if the thyroid gland is removed completely for carcinoma. *Tetany* is a classic feature of hypoparathyroidism, with numb-

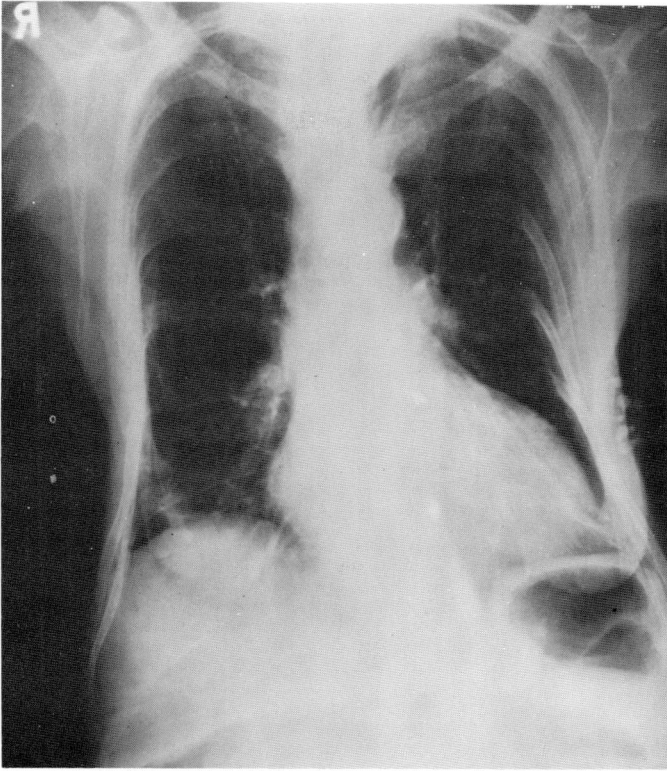

Fig. 3.22   Chest x-ray, showing rarefaction of all bones.

ness and tingling of the arms and legs, cramps, carpopedal spasm, laryngeal stridor, facial irritability and even convulsions. The total plasma calcium may fall to 1·5 mmol/litre (6 mg/100 ml). Phosphate rises to 1·9–3·8 mmol/litre (6–12 mg/100 ml).

Treatment. The initial treatment should be with 20 ml of 10 per cent calcium gluconate given slowly over 5–10 minutes. Calciferol 1·25 mg t.d.s. may be needed for long-term treatment, reducing the dose depending on the plasma calcium level (see p. 116).

References

Thyroid

Evered, D. C. (1976). Treatment of thyroid diseases. *British Medical Journal* **1,** 263 and 335.

Harvard, C. W. H. (1974a). Which test of thyroid function? *British Medical Journal* **1,** 553.

Harvard, C. W. H. (1974b). The management of thyrotoxicosis. *British Journal of Hospital Medicine* **11,** 893.

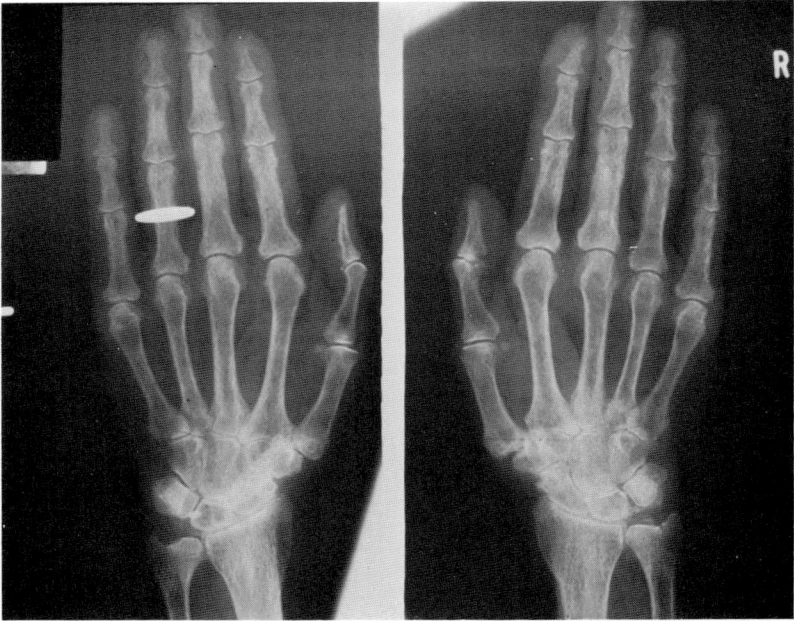

Fig. 3.23   Rarefaction of bones and subperiosteal erosions.

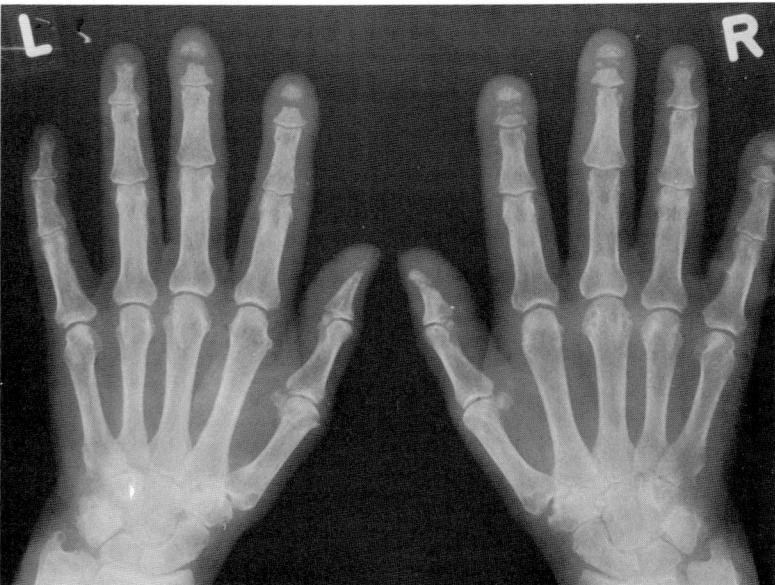

Fig. 3.24   Resorption of the terminal phalanges.

McConnon, J. K. (1973). The assessment of thyroid status. *British Journal of Hospital Medicine* **10**, 63.

McDevitt, H. (1977). Management of hyperthyroidism with beta blocking drugs. *Prescribers' Journal* **17**, 143.

Parathyroid

Tomlinson, S. and O'Riorden, J. M. H. (1978). The parathyroids. *British Journal of Hospital Medicine* **19**, 40.

Pituitary gland

The pituitary gland consists of two parts, an anterior and a posterior part, both under the control of the hypothalamus. The anterior pituitary lobe secretes seven hormones under the influence of stimuli from the hypothalamus. Thyroid-stimulating hormone (TSH) from the pituitary is stimulated by thyrotrophin-releasing hormone (TRH) from the hypothalamus, which in turn stimulates the thyroid gland. Corticotrophin from the hypothalamus stimulates secretion of adrenocorticotrophic hormone (ACTH), which stimulates the adrenal cortex. Other hormones released by the anterior pituitary under the influence of the hypothalamus include luteinizing hormone, follicular-stimulating hormone and interstitial cell-stimulating hormone (in man). Growth hormone is under the control of releasing factors and inhibiting factors from the hypothalamus. Prolactin may also be under dual control, as is the melanocyte-stimulating hormone. A variety of factors affect the hypothalamus, including stimuli from the appropriate target organs of the pituitary hormones.

In the anterior pituitary there are two types of cells: chromophobe and chromophil.

(1) Chromophobe: tumours of these cells rarely secrete and are associated with pressure on surrounding tissues, causing hypopituitarism.

(2) Chromophil cells are larger and may be divided into two groups—the eosinophils and the basophils. Over-secretion of the basophil cells gives rise to Cushing's disease, similar to Cushing's syndrome due to hyperfunction of the adrenal gland. Over-activity of the eosinophil cells gives rise to an excess of growth hormone, resulting in giantism and, in adult life, acromegaly.

In acromegaly the limbs are large, there is thickening of the skin and bones, the mandible, tongue, liver and heart are increased in size, sweating is common and hypertension is present. Diabetes may also be a feature. The thorax becomes stiff and kyphotic, and carpal tunnel syndrome may also be present. Because of the anatomical alterations in the jaw and tongue, intubation may be difficult and the tip of the Macintosh laryngoscope fails to visualize the larynx. The large tongue may lead to respiratory obstruction in the post-operative period. In addition, there may be neuromuscular complications (Picket *et al.*, 1975).

Prolactin

Prolactin is responsible for lactation. It is under the control of the hypothalamus. There is a prolactin-release-inhibiting hormone (PRIH) which may be dopamine. Phenothiazines and butyrophenones, which are dopamine antagonists, increase prolactin secretion (e.g. chlorpromazine, haloperodil) as do reserpine and α-methyldopa. Morphine, endorphin and oestrogens increase prolactin levels, as do stress and insulin-induced hypoglycaemia. Antiemetics (e.g. metoclopramide) also induce hyperprolactinaemia but bromocriptine, a dopamine agonist, restores the prolactin levels to normal (Besser *et al.*, 1977). Apomorphine and L-dopa reduce prolactin levels.

Hyperprolactinaemia is associated with infertility, amenorrhoea and galactorrhoea. Some pituitary tumours secrete excess prolactin even without galactorrhoea (Frantz, 1978). There have been suggestions that there is an association between the use of Rauwolfia and breast cancer (Armstrong *et al.*, 1974), and this is commented on by Morgan *et al.* (1976). Attention has also been drawn to the fact that prolactin levels rise during anaesthesia, especially with halothane (Cole *et al.*, 1976).

Hypopituitarism

Hypopituitarism is due to diminished activity of the pituitary gland, including ablation of the gland either by surgery or irradiation. The cause may be idiopathic or due to tumours, infection, fractures and cysts. In children, dwarfism results. Panhypopituitarism (Simmonds' disease) describes complete failure of the anterior pituitary gland, while Sheehan's syndrome was associated with acute blood loss in pregnancy resulting in infarction of the pituitary gland.

Hypopituitarism is associated with loss of hair, dryness and wrinkling of the skin, decreased sweating and pallor. There may be signs of adrenocortical insufficiency and hypothyroidism but aldosterone may still be secreted by the adrenal cortex.

Such patients are very sensitive to any form of stress such as injury, infection and the administration of sedatives. Coma may readily ensue with hypoglycaemia, hypothermia and loss of sodium with water intoxication. Underventilation is also a feature of the condition. The treatment of panhypopituitarism is to administer steroids (e.g. cortisone orally 25–37·5 mg per day). Thyroid hormone is often required in the dose of thyroxine 0·1–0·2 mg per day, but it should be given only when the patient is already on cortisone. The treatment of coma is to administer hydrocortisone 100 mg 4-hourly, 2·5–5 μg T_3 and intravenous glucose, with gradual rewarming if the patient is hypothermic.

For surgery to remove a chromophobe adenoma which is causing hypopituitarism, minimal anaesthetic agents are required and special care is required in the dosage of premedication and postoperative sedation. Intravenous hydrocortisone may be required during operation to prevent cardiovascular collapse.

Posterior pituitary gland

This is responsible for the production of antidiuretic hormone (ADH) and oxytocin. ADH (vasopressin) is unlike most of the other hormones secreted by cells of endocrine glands. The secretion comes from the supraoptic neurohypophyseal tract. The cell bodies are in the hypothalamus and the axon extends to the posterior lobe of the pituitary. Synthesis of vasopressin and oxytocin probably takes place in the cell body and they are stored in granules which move down to the posterior pituitary.

The main function of ADH is to increase water reabsorption in the distal tubule. The main stimuli for ADH release are blood volume depletion and a rise in plasma osmolality. Drugs such as morphine, pethidine and barbiturates stimulate the release of ADH, as does haemorrhage. Alcohol, phenytoin and glucocorticoids inhibit the release. Fentanyl is said to be one of the most powerful agents in releasing ADH (Bidwai *et al.*, 1976). Lithium used in the treatment of manic patients antagonizes the action of ADH.

ADH is also released by tumours such as bronchial oat-cell carcinoma, resulting in water retention and low sodium. This condition is referred to as the syndrome of inappropriate ADH secretion; it is also seen in brain injury, some lung diseases and after chlorpropamide.

Diabetes insipidus

This results from damage to the hypothalamic posterior pituitary axis. It may be idiopathic, associated with tumours in the pituitary gland, or may be due to metastases. The patients may have polyuria of the order of 4–20 litres per day. The urine is dilute with a low osmolality. Dehydration may ensue. Treatment involves the use of pitressin tannate 2·5–5 units by intramuscular injection. This has recently been replaced by a synthetic compound desmopressin (DDAVP). It can be given intravenously 10–20 μg once or twice a day or 1–4 μg by intramuscular injection per day. Solutions should not be diluted. This agent may have a place in the treatment of headache due to leakage of c.s.f. following spinal tap. Chlorothiazide is also effective in the treatment of diabetes insipidus in the dose of 50–150 mg per day, but the mode of action is not understood.

Surgery on the pituitary

Surgery is usually performed for pituitary tumour or the treatment of diabetes or carcinoma, particularly of the breast. This may be by direct surgical approach to the gland or by yttrium implant. Special points to note are that steroid and possible thyroid cover may be necessary as well as vasopressin for diabetes insipidus. In the latter case, dehydration may require fluid therapy. For carcinoma of the breast it is well to remember that there may be severe anaemia, pain in bone, pleural effusions and enlarged hilar glands with resulting superior vena cava obstruction. Fractures of bone are not uncommon in the presence of metastatic secondaries.

References

Armstrong, B., Stevens, N. *et al.* (1974). Retrospective study of the association between the use of rauwolfia derivatives and breast cancer in English women. *Lancet* **ii,** 672.

Besser, G. M., Thorner, M. O. *et al.* (1977). Absence of uterine neoplasia in patients on bromocriptine. *British Medical Journal* **2**, 868.

Bidwai, A. V., Liu, W. S. *et al.* (1976). The effects of large doses of fentanyl and fentanyl with nitrous oxide on renal function in the dog. *Canadian Anaesthetists' Society Journal* **23**, 296.

Cole, E. N., Holder, M. P. *et al.* (1976). Plasma-hormones during anaesthesia for breast surgery. *Lancet* **ii,** 1416.

Frantz, A. G. (1978). Prolactin. *New England Journal of Medicine* **298**, 201.

Morgan, L., Barrett, A. *et al.* (1976). Prolactin concentrations during anaesthesia. *British Medical Journal* **2**, 980.

Picket, A. B. E., Layzer, B. *et al.* (1975). Neuromuscular complications of acromegaly. *Neurology* **25**, 638.

Adrenal cortex

The adrenal cortex has three layers and these are, from without inwards, the zona glomerulosa, zona fasciculata and zona reticularis. Aldosterone is secreted by the zona glomerulosa whilst the other layers secrete glucocorticoids, androgens and some oestrogens and progesterones. Adrenocorticotrophic hormone (ACTH) influences the rate of secretion of glucocorticoids but has less effect on aldosterone.

Glucocorticoids

The principal glucocorticoids include cortisol (hydrocortisone) and corticosterone. The normal range of plasma cortisol is of the order of 200–700 nmol/litre (8–26 mcg/100 ml). Cholesterol is the precursor of most of the steroid hormones and the following represents the pathway of synthesis.

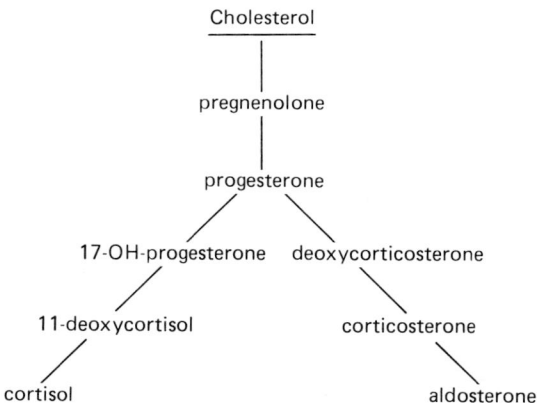

```
                          Cholesterol
                              |
                          pregnenolone
                              |
                          progesterone
                          /           \
        17-OH-progesterone       deoxycorticosterone
              /                            \
     11-deoxycortisol                 corticosterone
          /                                  \
     cortisol                            aldosterone
```

In addition, androgens and oestrogens are also formed. The corticosteroids are not stored in the adrenal gland and have to be synthesized in order to meet the normal body requirements. Secretion is regulated by ACTH which acts through the intermediary of cyclic AMP. ACTH causes the adrenal cortex to secrete cortisol, corticosteroids and, to some extent, aldosterone. Prolonged administration of ACTH results in hypertrophy of the adrenal cortex, while its absence causes the cortex to atrophy. There is a feedback mechanism by which raised cortisol levels inhibit the release of ACTH. If ACTH has to be given therapeutically it can be administered only by injection because it is destroyed in the gastrointestinal tract.

Cortisol is 90 per cent bound to plasma protein, initially to globulin and, when this is saturated, to albumin. Cortisol has a plasma half-life of about $1\frac{1}{2}$ hours; it is destroyed in the liver where it is initially reduced and then conjugated with glucuronic acid. The breakdown products are soluble and readily excreted. The duration of action of hydrocortisone (and ACTH) is approximately 6 hours.

Glucocorticoids affect carbohydrate, protein and lipid metabolism. They also affect electrolyte and water metabolism, muscle and blood, and modify the response to infection and trauma.

On carbohydrate and protein metabolism, glucocorticoids produce essentially catabolic effects. There is raised glucose production with hyperglycaemia and glycosuria. There is also increased liver glycogen, much of which comes from amino acids broken down from protein under the influence of cortisol. On lipid metabolism, cortisol increases the deposits of fat in the trunk while reducing it in the limbs. There is retention of sodium and excretion of potassium by the kidney: large amounts of cortisol cause sodium retention and increase in the extracellular water, leading to oedema. Cortisol is less effective in this respect than the naturally occurring mineralocorticoid, aldosterone. Steroids are necessary for the maintenance of skeletal muscle as weakness occurs in the absence of cortisol. However, in excessive doses, steroids give rise to myopathy. Cortisol depresses the development of cartilage and causes thinning of bone with osteoporosis.

Cortisol has an effect on the blood. It increases polymorphonuclear cells and the amount of haemoglobin, leading to polycythaemia, but depresses the number of lymphocytes and eosinophils. The metabolic response to injury or infection is suppressed. It has anti-inflammatory properties which may mask the signs of perforation of a peptic ulcer or promote the spread of infection.

Mineralocorticoids

The natural mineralocorticoid is aldosterone. It acts on the distal renal tubule and increases the absorption of sodium and the excretion of both potassium and hydrogen ions. Cortisol has similar effects but is less effective compared with aldosterone. Secretion of aldosterone is promoted when renin converts angiotensin 1 to angiotensin 2. Preparations of mineralocorticoids available include fludrocortisone and deoxycortone acetate.

Hyperfunction of the adrenal cortex

Cushing's syndrome is due to hyperactivity of the adrenal cortex. This may be ACTH-dependent due to excess secretion of ACTH from the pituitary gland (Cushing's disease), from the administration of ACTH or from tumours of non-endocrine origin which secrete ACTH.

Cushing's syndrome may be non-ACTH-dependent due to the administration of steroids or due to adenoma or carcinoma of the adrenal cortex. In some instances one adrenal may be active and the other atrophic. At operation to remove the hypertrophic adrenal gland, replacement therapy is indicated, otherwise signs of adrenal hypofunction will readily ensue.

Congenital adrenal hyperplasia may result in adrenal insufficiency because of defective enzymes capable of synthesizing glucocorticoids. This results in a negative feedback to the pituitary, which secretes ACTH and stimulates the adrenal to produce an excess of androgens.

The signs of adrenal hyperfunction include obesity, moonface, striae on the skin of the abdomen, weakness, osteoporosis, kyphosis, alkalosis, hypokalaemia, diabetes and hypertension. Hirsutism and menstrual disorders are often present, depending on the type of steroid that an adrenal tumour is secreting.

Cushing's syndrome may be due to carcinoma of the lung secreting ACTH in large quantities. Features of this condition include alkalosis, loss of potassium and pigmentation. Hypertension and moonface are seldom seen because the disease is rapidly fatal.

Diagnosis

The diagnosis of overactivity of the adrenal cortex can be made by the following measurements.

(1) Plasma cortisone levels (when interpreting these results, one must bear in mind that there are diurnal variations).
(2) Suppression of cortisol production by oral steroids.
(3) Administration of radioactive cortisol and measuring metabolites.
(4) Radioimmunoassay of plasma ACTH.
(5) Adrenal androgen can be assessed by measuring urinary 17-ketosteroids.

Treatment

Cushing's disease is best treated by interfering with the production of ACTH from the pituitary. The pituitary may be approached surgically, irradiated or destroyed by implantation of radioactive yttrium. Better results are obtained with bilateral adrenalectomy and irradiation. Adrenalectomy with irradiation results in enlargement of the pituitary fossa, with possible pressure on the optic chiasma and possible pigmentation. Cushing's syndrome due to excessive treatment with ACTH or corticosteroids should indicate the need to carefully reduce the dose of these drugs. During surgery and following operation full steroid cover will be necessary; in addition, the mineralocorticoid, fludrocortisone, 0·1 mg per day will be required. During operation care should be taken not to overload the circulation with saline and to bear in mind the problems associated with alkalosis and hypokalaemia. In the latter case non-depolarizing relaxants may have a prolonged action. The hypertension may present problems and drugs should be given slowly to avoid rapid changes in blood pressure. Myocardial-depressant drugs, intermittent positive pressure ventilation and muscle relaxants (tubocurarine, which can cause ganglion blockade) readily produce hypotension. Intubation may be difficult because of the moonface; ventilation pressures need to be adjusted to cope with the obesity and the restriction of ventilation due to kyphosis. The osteoporosis should not be forgotten, as injudicious handling of the patient could result in fractures. In the postoperative phase a high-protein diet, potassium chloride and testosterone may be required in addition to the steroid cover (glucocorticoid and mineralocorticoid).

Miscellaneous drugs

Mitotane is a drug very similar in structure to the insecticide DDT and it destroys selectively the cells of the adrenal cortex whether they be normal or malignant. Nausea and vomiting are frequent with its use, but it is of value in carcinoma of the adrenal gland.

Aminoglutethimide compound inhibits the first stage of steroid synthesis from cholesterol, and therefore interrupts both cortisol and aldosterone production. It is not suitable for hyperfunction of the adrenal which is ACTH-dependent. Fall in circulating cortisol leads to further secretion of ACTH, which again raises the level of cortisol.

Metyrapone. This compound blocks the production of cortisol by inhibiting the enzyme 11β-hydroxylase activity which is needed to produce cortisol from its immediate precursor, 11-deoxycortisol. Aldosterone is unaffected. Metyrapone is of value in the long-term management of Cushing's disease or in carcinoma of the adrenal gland. In the preparation of patients for surgery with adrenocortical adenoma, metyrapone is of value in controlling many of the features of adrenal hyperplasia such as hypertension, diabetes and obesity. Operative morbidity may therefore be reduced (Besser and Jeffcoate, 1976). It is not suitable for pituitary-dependent adrenal hypersecretion because it inhibits the production of cortisone, which in turn leads to an increase in ACTH production.

Adrenal cortex hypofunction

The first description of this condition was given by Addison in 1855, and the disease now bears his name. Observations were followed up in 1856 by Brown-Séquard, who removed the adrenal glands in animals and noted their necessity for survival. Adrenocortical failure may be (1) primary or (2) secondary due to lack of ACTH.

Primary

Primary adrenocortical failure may be due to autoimmune disease, tuberculosis, amyloid disease or metastatic carcinoma in the adrenal gland. Idiopathic adrenal failure is now believed to be due to autoimmune disease, as there are antibodies in the serum. It may be suspected when there are other autoimmune diseases associated with it such as thyroid failure, anaemia, ovarian dysfunction and diabetes.

Other causes include bilateral adrenalectomy for carcinoma of the breast or for adrenal disease, or Cushing's disease. The adrenals may be damaged at operation, become infarcted, or suffer intracapsular haemorrhage. Adrenal failure may occur in overwhelming infection (Waterhouse–Friderichsen syndrome).

Secondary

Secondary adrenocortical failure may be due to hypopituitarism, pituitary tumours, hypothalamic trauma or encephalitis. Corticosteroids used for adrenal suppression, for collagen disease, blood disorders or prior to transplant surgery may likewise suppress adrenal function. Congenital adrenal hyperplasia may result in reduced glucocorticoid activity.

Signs of adrenal insufficiency

Adrenal insufficiency may be chronic (Addison's disease) or acute (adrenal crisis).

Chronic insufficiency (Addison's disease)

Addison's disease, in which the whole of the adrenal gland is destroyed, results in insufficiency of cortisol and aldosterone production. The features are weakness, loss of weight, hypotension, pigmentation and symptoms similar to those of gastroenteritis. Abdominal pain may be mistaken for appendicitis. Pigmentation affects not only the exposed skin but also the mucous membrane of both mouth and conjunctiva. Hypoglycaemia may be present, the hair may be lost and menstrual disorders are not uncommon. Patients are particularly sensitive to sedation, infection and insulin. There is a decrease in reabsorption of sodium and chloride by the kidney and a rise in the plasma potassium. Eventually dehydration ensues with a reduction in blood pressure and renal blood flow. Nausea and vomiting further increase dehydration.

Pigmentation is often the first sign of reduced adrenal activity. For example, a patient with a preoperative systolic blood pressure of 130 mmHg had a hernia repair. He was premedicated with morphine and atropine, and anaesthesia consisted of thiopentone, suxamethonium, tubocurarine, nitrous oxide and oxygen. During operation the blood pressure fell to 80 mmHg systolic and, despite intravenous therapy and vasopressors, it did not rise above 90 mmHg systolic. The patient remained perfectly well apart from a slight degree of lassitude and a blood pressure between 90 and 100 mmHg for three months after operation, when pigmentation of the skin appeared—suggesting the diagnosis of Addison's disease (personal communication).

Acute insufficiency

This occurs when the adrenals are incapable of responding to the stress of infection, trauma or operation. There is profound hypotension, muscular weakness, oliguria, hypothermia and vomiting. The sodium loss is greater than water loss, resulting in a decrease in osmotic pressure of the extracellular fluid. Excess water enters the cells, producing water intoxication. The plasma potassium is raised as well as the plasma urea. Initially the temperature may be raised, but this is followed by hypothermia.

Tests for adrenocortical insufficiency

These include:

(1) measurement of the plasma electrolytes;
(2) measurement of plasma cortisol levels, allowing for diurnal variations;
(3) the response to ACTH stimulation;
(4) the cautious use of the insulin-induced hypoglycaemic test;
(5) metyrapone test for assessing hypothalamus–pituitary function;
(6) ACTH levels in the plasma.

Treatment

Chronic adrenal insufficiency. With destruction of the adrenal gland both glucocorticoid and mineralocorticoid steroid hormones will be necessary. However, in ACTH deficiency the secretion of aldosterone is unaffected. Cortisone acetate by mouth has been used routinely in the dose of 25 mg in the morning and 12·5 mg in the evening. The disadvantage of this agent is that it has to be converted in the liver to hydrocortisone (cortisol). This treatment is being replaced by hydrocortisone, 20 mg in the morning and 10 mg in the evening. The correct dose can be assessed by measuring plasma cortisol levels throughout the day. Synthetic steroids may be used instead: prednisolone 5 and 2·5 mg or dexamethasone 0·5 and 0·25 mg (see Table 3.4). These doses may need to be increased if infection occurs, while any gastrointestinal upset with vomiting requires intramuscular injection of hydrocortisone.

Table 3.4 Preparations of glucocorticoids available and their relative potencies. (Adapted from Baird and Strong, 1977)

Cortisol	1	Triamcinolone	5
Cortisone	0·8	Betamethasone	25
Prednisone	4	Dexamethasone	25
Prednisolone	4		

Prednisone and prednisolone have some effect on sodium retention while betamethasone and dexamethasone have none.

To replace the loss of aldosterone, fludrocortisone is required in the dose of 0·05–0·1 mg either daily or on alternate days. Alternative preparations to fludrocortisone include deoxycortone acetate (DOCA) or deoxycortone trimethylacetate (DCTMA) which is a long-acting compound (0·1 mg of fludrocortisone equals 2·5 mg of DOCA equals 75 mg DCTMA).

Acute adrenal insufficiency. This requires intravenous fluid to correct the peripheral circulatory failure and the dehydration. Five per cent dextrose is necessary to correct hypoglycaemia, and saline to correct the sodium loss. Hydrocortisone hemisuccinate should be given intravenously 100 mg every 6 hours. Pressor amines are not of much value. Five litres of intravenous fluid may be required in the first 24 hours, and if the crisis is precipitated by infection, suitable antibiotics should be administered. Intramuscular injections of 10 mg of deoxycortone acetate should be given twice in the first 24 hours. The patient's blood pressure, e.c.g. and central venous pressure should be monitored.

Therapy with steroids

Apart from their use in replacement therapy, steroids are of value in the suppression of autoimmune states and allergic responses. The dose required is much greater than the daily requirements of the patient. Steroids can be used in the treatment of the following conditions.

Arthritis, either by oral preparation or by injection into painful joints.
In renal disease—the nephrotic syndrome.
Diseases of the connective tissue, except scleroderma which is resistant.
Polymyositis, polyarteritis nodosa, giant cell arteritis and systemic lupus erythematosus.
Allergic states—hay fever, urticaria, dermatitis, angioneurotic oedema and anaphylactic shock.
Asthma—hydrocortisone in the treatment of status asthmaticus; chronic asthmatics benefit from oral therapy.
Sarcoidosis: there is thickening of the membrane in the lung, preventing the rapid transfer of oxygen; steroids have a beneficial effect on the lung membrane in the early stages of the disease.
Inflammatory conditions of the eye respond to local treatment.
Various skin disorders respond to steroid therapy applied locally, but prolonged treatment gives rise to atrophy of the skin.
Chronic ulcerative colitis may have the symptoms alleviated.
Myasthenia gravis: prednisone is recommended for those patients who are not well controlled with anticholinesterases, after thymectomy and in older males; the initial dose should not be greater than 25 mg, otherwise weakness may occur (Drachman, 1978).
Leukaemia, lymphoma, thrombocytopenia, haemolytic anaemia.
Hepatitis.
Organ transplantation: steroids are used to suppress rejection phenomena.

The following conditions are of particular interest to anaesthetists:

(1) patients with cerebral oedema;
(2) shock;
(3) aspiration of gastric contents.

Cerebral oedema

Patients with cerebral oedema from brain trauma, brain tumour and those with raised intracranial pressure respond to steroid therapy, especially with dexamethasone. The initial dose is 10 mg intravenously followed by 4 mg intramuscularly every 6 hours. Palliative therapy with steroids in a reduced dosage may be effective.

Shock

The evidence in favour of massive doses of steroids in the treatment of shock is conflicting (Reichgott and Melmon, 1973). It has been recommended in endotoxic shock and overwhelming bacteraemic shock. Haemorrhagic and cardiogenic shock should be treated with appropriate measures such as fluid replacement, with electrolytes, antibiotics and plasma volume expanders. Steroids have been recommended as an adjunct to therapy when all routine methods of treatment appear to have failed. The rationale for their use stems from the fact that in endotoxic shock the adrenals may suffer haemorrhage and steroids are required. It has been claimed that pressor amines fail to work without an adequate supply of steroids; but steroids are vasodilators and therefore improve tissue perfusion and are believed to antagonize the vasoconstrictor effects of pressor amines. The recommended dose is dexamethasone 2–6 mg/kg body weight intravenously, repeated after 2–6 hours.

Aspiration of gastric contents

Aspiration of gastric contents entering the bronchial tract results in pulmonary oedema (Mendelson's syndrome). Massive doses of steroids have been recommended in the dose of 100 mg hydrocortisone intravenously 6-hourly. Recently Wolf et al. (1977) have shown that steroids do not decrease the overall mortality. They appear to suppress the response in the lung, with the result that Po_2 does not drop markedly and the x-ray appearance shows less damage. Direct instillation of steroids into the lung via an endotracheal tube is not recommended. The one disturbing aspect of this therapy is that after a period of five days the incidence of E-coli pneumonia is increased. Overall mortality between those treated with steroids and the untreated was not significantly different.

Hazards associated with steroid therapy

Patients on replacement therapy with steroids. This group are particularly at risk from infection, trauma and surgery, when their steroid requirements may increase.

Patients on large doses of steroids for immunosuppressive therapy. Side effects may be divided into (1) metabolic and (2) suppression of adrenal secretion. The metabolic disturbances include sodium and fluid retention, congestive cardiac failure, hypokalaemic alkalosis, moonface, obesity and diabetes. There is said to be an increase in incidence of thromboembolism. Electrolyte disturbances are less likely with triamcinolone and dexamethasone. There is an increased susceptibility to infection, especially tuberculosis and fungal infections. Patients on steroids should not be vaccinated. In addition, cataracts can occur on prolonged therapy, and osteoporosis and collapse of vertebrae are not infrequent—especially in postmenopausal women. Proximal myopathies occasionally occur; psychiatric disturbances are reported, ranging from severe depression and psychotic disturbances to personality change, insomnia and suicidal tendencies. Often during steroid therapy patients have a sense of euphoria, only to fall in fits of depression when the therapy is stopped. Peptic ulceration with haemorrhage has been reported to be more frequent in patients on steroid therapy. The evidence for this is less clear cut than had been formerly supposed. Many of the episodes have been reported in patients with rheumatoid arthritis in whom gastric acid secretion is higher than the rest of the population, and yet other drugs such as aspirin have frequently been taken as well. Until the evidence is more clear cut, steroids should be given with great care in patients with a history of an ulcer (Douglas, 1977).

Other relative contraindications to steroid therapy are renal insufficiency and diverticulitis (when a diverticulum may perforate).

Suppression of the hypophyseal pituitary axis is revealed when steroids are withdrawn from patients on large continuous doses. This renders the patients just as susceptible as those with adrenocortical insufficiency to stress situations. Patients should preferably be weaned from steroid therapy gradually, taking care in case ACTH therapy may also be necessary to compensate for the pituitary suppression.

Suppression of adrenocortical function may occur when steroids are given topically or even rectally. Patients on steroid therapy may develop adrenal failure if barbiturates are given for sedation. Phenobarbitone is known to produce enzyme induction which stimulates the liver microsomes to accelerate the rate of destruction of substances normally destroyed in the liver (e.g. steroids).

Steroid therapy and surgery

Many regimens have been proposed for the management of patients undergoing surgery during the course of steroid therapy. Strong (1978) recommended that 100 mg cortisone acetate should be given the night before operation, with 200 mg on the morning of operation and repeated in doses of 50 mg 6-hourly in the postoperative period. After 24 hours, routine maintenance therapy is possible. For adrenalectomy, larger doses are required; namely, 200 mg per day, tailing off to the maintenance dose of 37·5 mg over a period of days.

Many of the regimens proposed for surgery were based on the fact that, originally, the initial preparation of cortisone (which was in alcoholic solution) had to be diluted in a large volume of fluid before it could be administered. Furthermore, the fact that cortisone was the only preparation available meant that it had to be converted in the liver to hydrocortisone (cortisol) before it could be effective. The introduction of soluble preparations of hydrocortisone–hydrocortisone hemisuccinate altered the need for complicated regimens of treatment.

Plumpton *et al.* (1969a) showed that there was a rise in plasma cortisol levels during surgery which was in relationship to the severity of the surgery irrespective of whether they were normal patients or those who had had steroid therapy but were no longer under treatment. It was shown that adrenocortical suppression was very unlikely to be present two months after treatment had been withdrawn. With patients on steroid therapy, they could find no clear relationship between the dose and duration of steroid therapy and the ability to respond to surgery. In a subsequent paper, Plumpton *et al.* (1969b) showed that in 20 patients who were known to have an inadequate adrenocortical response to stress as assessed by insulin hypoglycaemic test, that intramuscular hydrocortisone hemisuccinate 100 mg 6-hourly for at least three days produced adequate cover for major surgery. Steroid treatment started with premedication. For intermediate operations such as inguinal hernia, 24 hours' cover was deemed to be adequate, while for short diagnostic procedures one dose was sufficient. In the postoperative phase, they recommended that steroids be stopped abruptly because there was no real evidence to show that gradual reduction of the dose was beneficial. If anything, abrupt cessation of steroid cover would produce the maximum stimulation of the hypophyseal pituitary adrenal axis. These recommendations are based on the assumption that no complications have ensued. However, requirements must be increased should infection occur. It is advisable to administer anaesthetic agents and analgesics with care. Unexplained hypotension during operation is readily treated with the intravenous injection of 100 mg of hydrocortisone hemisuccinate.

Aldosterone

Hypersecretion of aldosterone may be primary or secondary. *Primary* aldosteronism is often associated with adenoma (Conn's syndrome) or hyperplasia. *Secondary* aldosteronism occurs in cirrhosis of the liver, in nephrotic syndrome and in severe cardiac failure. Renin-secreting tumours of the kidney or renal artery stenosis are also causes and may be amenable to surgical treatment.

Aldosterone acts on the distal renal tubule, promoting the reabsorption of sodium and the excretion of potassium and hydrogen ions. The diagnosis of hypersecretion of aldosterone is characterized by weakness, thought to be due to potassium deficiency. There is metabolic alkalosis and, often, tetany. The blood pressure is raised, with sodium retention and potassium loss.

Increased secretion of aldosterone occurs with a low sodium intake, dehydration, increased potassium intake and haemorrhage. Decreased secretion occurs with a high salt intake, a reduced potassium intake and an increased extracellular volume. Aldosterone has no effect on the secretion of ACTH. A lack of aldosterone leads to sodium loss, potassium retention, dehydration and hypotension.

Surgery

Adrenal adenoma, which may be bilateral, is amenable to surgical treatment. In view of the attendant dangers of low potassium, it is advisable to prepare the patient with an antagonist. Spironolactone, an analogue of aldosterone, is a competitive antagonist to it. Spironolactone (Aldactone) is given orally in the dose of 100–400 mg per day until the level of potassium is controlled. Supplement of potassium may also be necessary. After removal of the tumour, there may be rebound phenomena in which there is hyperkalaemia, necessitating the use of fludrocortisone for a short period of time. Spironolactone may be necessary for those patients who are not suitable for surgery.

References

Baird, J. D. and Strong, J. A. (1977). Endocrines and metabolic diseases. In: *Davidson's Principles and Practice of Medicine*, p. 549. Ed. by J. MacLeod. Churchill Livingstone, Edinburgh and London.

Besser, G. M. and Jeffcoate, W. J. (1976). Endocrine and metabolic diseases—adrenal diseases. *British Medical Journal* **1**, 448.

Douglas, A. P. (1977). *Textbook of Adverse Drug Reactions*, p. 139. Ed. by D. M. Davies. Oxford University Press, Oxford.

Drachman, D. B. (1978). Myasthenia gravis. *New England Journal of Medicine* **298**, 186.

Plumpton, F. S., Besser, G. M. *et al.* (1969a). Corticosteroid treatment and surgery—an investigation of indications of steroid cover. *Anaesthesia* **24**, 3.

Plumpton, F. S., Besser, G. M. *et al.* (1969b). Corticosteroid treatment and surgery—the management of steroid cover. *Anaesthesia* **24**, 12.

Reichgott, M. G. and Melmon, K. L. (1973). Should corticosteroids be used in shock? *Medical Clinics of North America* **57**, 1211.

Strong, J. A. (1978). *Textbook of Medical Treatment*, 14th edn, p. 239. Ed. by S. Alstead and R. H. Girdwood. Churchill Livingstone, Edinburgh and London.

Wolf, J. E., Bone, R. C. *et al.* (1977). Effects of corticosteroids in the treatment of patients with gastric aspiration. *American Journal of Medicine* **63**, 719.

Carcinoid tumours

Carcinoid tumours appear in plaques just under the mucosa in the gastrointestinal tract. The tumours are also known as argentaffinomas because the cells reduce silver salts. In 1953 Lembeck extracted 5-hydroxytryptamine (5-HT; serotonin) from a carcinoid tumour.

The characteristics of the carcinoid syndrome are: (1) vasomotor, (2) gastrointestinal and (3) cardiorespiratory.

The vasomotor symptoms consist of cutaneous flushing of the face and neck which go from red to white, and facial and periorbital oedema. Precipitating factors include food, alcohol, emotion, physical activity, manipulation of the tumour and the administration of intravenous pressor amines.

The gastrointestinal symptoms are discomfort, diarrhoea, pain from secondaries, hepatomegaly and ascites.

The cardiorespiratory symptoms are reduced blood pressure, tachycardia, right-sided heart failure, oedema and bronchospasm. In addition, there may be nutritional deficiencies, including weight loss, reduced serum albumin and pellagra.

The tumours often occur in the appendix, ileum or jejunum. The tumour metastasizes to the lymph nodes, liver and other organs via the blood vessels, and occurs in about 30 per cent of patients. Only about 25 per cent of patients with carcinoid tumour have symptoms due to the secretion of serotonin and other vasoactive agents. Bronchial adenoma may also secrete vasoactive substances.

5-Hydroxytryptamine

In the adult, about 95 per cent of the total body serotonin (5-HT) is in the chromaffin cells of the gastrointestinal tract, with the remainder in the platelets, brain and spleen.

5-Hydroxytryptamine (5-HT) is produced from tryptophan which is hydroxylated to form 5-hydroxytryptophan (5-HTP). After decarboxylation, 5-HT is formed. Most of the 5-HT is destroyed in the liver by monoaminoxidase to form 5-hydroxyacetaldehyde. This is further oxidized to 5-hydroxyindole acetic acid (5-HIAA) which is excreted in the urine (Fig. 3.25). The diagnosis of carcinoid syndrome may be made on the excretion of 5-HIAA; normally 2–9 mg per day is present in the urine but in carcinoid syndrome this is increased to 50–600 mg per day. There is about 10 mg of 5-HT in the human body and it appears that the amount equal to this is synthesized every day, but with carcinoid tumour this would increase to 50–600 mg/day. Tryptophan, in addition to forming 5-HT is necessary for the production of niacin and nicotinic acid. In carcinoid syndrome, 60 times more 5-HT may be produced, causing a deficiency of nicotinic acid—which results in pellagra.

The function of 5-HT is still speculative, even though it has diverse effects on the following systems.

Respiratory system

The respiratory effects of 5-HT vary according to the animals studied, but

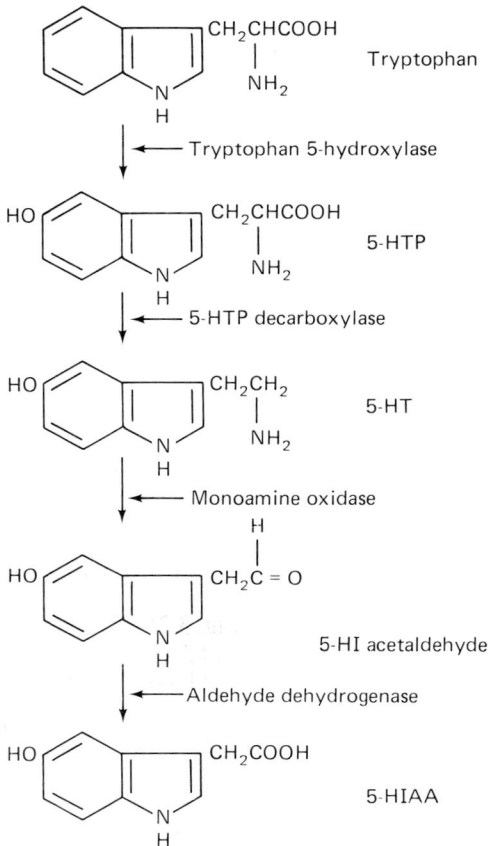

Fig. 3.25   The carcinoid syndrome.

in man hyperpnoea occurs with increased bronchiolar tone, especially in the asthmatic subject.

Cardiovascular system

The cardiovascular effects of 5-HT are complex, producing vasoconstriction especially in the kidney. It dilates the blood vessels in muscles and in the skin, but also produces vasoconstriction of the arterioles in the skin. The veins are also constricted. Cardiac output is increased with stimulation of the rate and force of the heart. In man, the blood pressure initially falls; this is succeeded by an increase in blood pressure and finally there is a prolonged fall in blood pressure. These complex responses are due to reflexes, effects of baroreceptor stimulation, while the late prolonged fall in blood pressure is said to be due to dilatation in the skeletal muscles.

   In the carcinoid syndrome, fibrous tissue is laid down in the endocardium of the chambers of the heart and the cusps. Pulmonary stenosis, tricuspid stenosis and regurgitation are reported. This may be due to the effect of 5-HT, as it has been shown to increase fibroblastic activity.

Alimentary tract

This is stimulated by 5-HT, resulting in intense spasm followed by increased contractions, and finally inhibition. It is also possible that it may be a transmitter in the gut muscle contraction.

Central nervous system

5-HT is now believed to be a transmitter but its exact role is still undetermined. It appears to be involved in depressing exaggerated responses to stimuli. It affects mood, behaviour, aggression and sleep (REM). Lysergide (LSD) reduces the 5-HT turnover in the brain.

Features

Some of the signs and symptoms of carcinoid syndrome are not entirely explained by the actions of 5-HT. These may be due to the effect of plasma kinins. The two most commonly implicated are kallikrein (Greek for *pancreas*, which contains this material) and bradykinin (Greek for slow acting on *bowel*). These substances are vasoactive polypeptides and only become active when released from their precursors. They are released by changes of pH, temperature, contact with glass and damage to tissues. Factor XII is also involved. Kinins are very rapidly broken down in the plasma. Their role in the production of carcinoid syndrome is still not completely understood but inhibitors are recommended in the treatment of the symptoms of carcinoid syndrome.

Drugs

Many drugs have been recommended in the treatment of patients with symptoms of carcinoid syndrome, but none seems entirely successful in view of the widespread effects of 5-HT and doubts whether this agent produces all the symptoms. Steroids, ε-aminocaproic acid and aprotinin have been advocated in inhibiting the release of kinins. Drugs which antagonize 5-HT include antihistamines, phenothiazines especially chlorpromazine and methotrimeprazine, methysergide, cyproheptadine, parachlorphenylalanine and adrenergic-blocking agents (e.g. phenoxybenzamine).

Other drugs affecting 5-HT are: reserpine, which releases it; tricyclics, which prevent the uptake of 5-HT by platelets; and methyldopa, which inhibits the conversion of 5-HTP to 5-HT. Parachlorphenylalanine only affects the diarrhoea and has too many side effects to be used clinically; it inhibits the conversion of tryptophan to 5-HTP. Methysergide, which is closely related to LSD, takes 1–2 days to act and affects mostly the diarrhoea; the side effects are numerous, including gastrointestinal disturbances, insomnia, confusion, excitement and hallucinations. Cyproheptadine is a powerful antihistamine, and one of its side effects is drowsiness.

Anaesthesia

Anaesthesia in carcinoid syndrome may be required for surgical removal of tumour, or may be for other operations in the presence of carcinoid. 5-HT is normally destroyed in the liver by amine oxidase, and it is believed only to cause symptoms when the liver is unable to handle the excess of 5-HT.

The hazards which occur at operation are usually bronchospasm, hypotension, hypertension and tachycardia, facial flushing and even oedema. Mason and Steane (1976) have suggested the following programme of management. Aprotinin 200 000 units should be given 1 hour before surgery and continued 4-hourly, if it is believed that kinins are involved in causing symptoms. Morphine is considered inadvisable because it might release 5-HT; suxamethonium might cause compression of the tumour, whilst *d*-tubocurarine, gallamine and alcuronium may have effects on blood pressure. Pancuronium is recommended as the muscle relaxant of choice. Vasopressors are not recommended because they might release kinins. Close monitoring of the patient is advised. Delayed recovery may occur after anaesthesia in carcinoid syndrome because of the central effects of 5-HT. Bronchospasm may be relieved by intravenous aminophylline, hydrocortisone or aerosols of sympathomimetic agents which are contraindicated if given intravenously (Turck *et al.*, 1972).

Mason and Steane (1976) reported the management of one patient in detail. Their patient was prepared with oral cyproheptadine 4 mg t.d.s. for two days before operation, 4 mg on the morning of operation and 4 mg with premedication. Premedication was with pethidine and atropine. Anaesthesia consisted of thiopentone, fentanyl, pancuronium, nitrous oxide and oxygen, and ventilation was controlled with increments of fentanyl and pancuronium. Aprotinin was not used. At operation the blood pressure rose to 160–170 mmHg. The small bowel had increased peristalsis and the blood glucose rose to 12·5 mmol/litre (225 mg/100 ml). Two doses of 2·5 mg of methotrimeprazine given intravenously reduced the peristalsis in the small intestine and controlled the rise in blood pressure. Postoperatively 10 mg of pethidine produced excessive drowsiness.

References

Mason, R. A. and Steane, P. A. (1976). Carcinoid syndrome, its relevance to the anaesthetist. *Anaesthesia* **31**, 228.
Turck, W. P. G., Zeitlin, I. J. *et al.* (1972). Airways obstruction investigation of reversible airways obstruction. *Scottish Medical Journal* **17**, 237.

4

Anaemia

Anaemia may be defined in functional or pathological terms. However, the pathological definition of anaemia as a lowering of the concentration of haemoglobin (Hb) in the blood below the normal range for the age and sex of the patient as measured in a particular laboratory, does not take into account changes which may take place in the plasma volume or the concentration of Hb in each red cell.

Because the concentration of Hb is not the sole determinant of oxygen delivery to the tissues, the pathological definition is incomplete and the functional definition is better—'a reduction in the oxygen-transporting and tissue-oxygenating capacity of the blood'. The physiological consequences of anaemia depend on both the concentration of Hb and the oxygen affinity of Hb, and though primary changes in the latter are unusual, oxygen affinity is under the influence of such factors as pH, temperature, mean cell haemoglobin concentration and, possibly most important, the 2,3-diphosphoglycerate (2,3-DPG) concentration in the red cells.

Classification of anaemias (Brain, 1975)

The common classification of anaemias is according to the *aetiology*.

(1) Principally caused by impaired production of red cells:
   (a) at stem cell level
       e.g. aplastic anaemia; chronic renal failure;
   (b) disturbances of proliferation and maturation of differential erythroblasts
       e.g. iron deficiency; B_{12}, folic acid deficiency; marrow infiltrations.
(2) Shortened red cell survival:
   (a) red cell abnormalities
       e.g. sickle cell disease; spherocytosis;
   (b) extrinsic factors:
       e.g. splenomegaly; toxic agents; bacterial agents.
(3) Anaemia of blood loss (acute or chronic).

An alternative classification is based on the *microscopic appearance* of the red cells.

(1) Macrocytic (mean cell volume more than 94 μm^3), e.g. B_{12} deficiency.
(2) Normocytic, e.g. acute blood loss or with chronic disease.
(3) Microcytic and hypochromic (mean cell haemoglobin concentrations less than 32 per cent).

Renal failure is usually accompanied by a severe anaemia. Degrees of elevation of the blood urea parallel the decreased red cell life span. Patients on haemodialysis lose iron with blood in the dialysis coil, and folate is also removed by dialysis. Progressive disease of kidneys leads to decreased erythropoietin production and, in addition, the marrow's response may be reduced by the uraemia. One of the reasons why patients with chronic renal failure on dialysis survive with very low haemoglobin levels is that the oxygen dissociation curve shifts to the right under the influence of an increased red cell 2,3-DPG (see below). Also, compensations occur within the cardiovascular system, as they do with any anaemia.

The normal response to increased demand by the tissues for oxygen is met by an increase in cardiac output and so the symptoms of anaemia first present on exercise or in other situations demanding an increase in cardiac output. Patients with severe anaemia are dyspnoeic on exertion or even at rest. There occurs an increase in cardiac output in an attempt to increase tissue perfusion, with the result that flow murmurs may be audible in the young and there may be manifestations of congestive cardiac failure in the elderly. The elderly myocardium suffers also from fatty infiltration in chronic anaemia (especially B_{12} deficiency) and its function may already be reduced by hypoxia associated with the low haemoglobin. Anaemic patients also have an increased alveolar–arterial oxygen difference ($A-aDo_2$) at rest.

Nunn (1969) introduced the concept of oxygen 'flux', which is the quantity of oxygen delivered to the tissues each minute.

$$O_2 \text{ flux} = \text{ml } O_2 \text{ carried by 1 g of Hb} =$$
$$\text{cardiac output} \times \frac{\text{Hb saturation}\%}{100} \times 1\cdot39 \text{ ml/g} \times \text{Hb conc.}$$

($1\cdot39$ is a constant related to the molecular weight of haemoglobin.)

Tissue oxygenation must depend on cardiac output and arterial oxygen saturation so, with good cardiac and pulmonary function, the Hb concentration can be reduced without necessarily reducing tissue oxygenation, though there will be less reserve.

A large quantity of oxygen remains in venous blood (70 per cent saturation) and this is a readily available store which can be called upon without increasing the cardiac output. However, any reduction in venous oxygen content which occurs when the oxygen flux is reduced must lower the venous Po_2. This in turn causes a reduction in the tissue Po_2 by lowering the head of pressure for diffusion of oxygen into the tissues.

However, it is acknowledged that anaesthesia can be administered, without obvious detriment, to patients with Hb levels chronically as low as 6 g/dl (such levels as are commonly seen in patients with chronic renal failure) (Gillies, 1974). Tissue oxygenation at these levels is maintained by hyper-fusion of essential organs by a raised cardiac output where this is possible. Shifts in the oxygen dissociation curve to the right also help to compensate. In work done on experimental animals, Cullen and Eger (1970) found no biochemical evidence of tissue hypoxia after reduction of the haematocrit to 10 per cent; but loss of red cell mass may lead to decreased tissue oxygenation only partially compensated for by adjustments in cardiovascular dynamics.

Treatment

Principles of the treatment of anaemia must always depend on the recognition of the cause. Iron therapy, for example, should be given only when the anaemia is shown to be caused by iron deficiency, because of inadequate intake or increased demand (as in pregnancy). When 10 per cent of the circulating blood volume has been lost acutely, half of the red cells and plasma is replaced by plasma alone after 24 hours. When 20 per cent is lost, it takes 24–60 hours to replace the circulatory volume.

World wide, iron deficiency anaemia is the commonest type and exists when the mean cell Hb concentration is less than 30 per cent and hypochromia exists on the blood film. When iron therapy is indicated, a total daily dose of iron of 180–240 mg orally should give maximal rates of Hb regeneration in adults. Organic ferrous compounds usually cause less intestinal disturbance but ferrous sulphate 60 mg 8-hourly is often satisfactory. The oral doses for infants start at 60–90 mg daily and rise rapidly for older children, who may be given adult doses.

Parenteral iron is a rapid and effective method when a calculated dose should be given in either intravenous or intramuscular form. Each 25 mg of iron raises the Hb level by 0·15 g/dl; therefore the dose given should be the calculated amount necessary to raise the Hb to normal levels, plus 500 mg to replenish iron stores.

Great care should be exercised if anaemia is to be treated with blood transfusion. The myocardium is probably already under stress and extra circulating blood volume may precipitate congestive cardiac failure. Small volumes are needed, preferably of packed cells of fresh citrate phosphate dextrose (CPD) blood and, in addition, the use of diuretics should be considered.

The total volume of blood necessary to transfuse a patient is roughly calculated from the formula:

$$\text{Volume of transfused blood} = \frac{\text{normal blood volume} \times \text{Hb\%/dl rise needed}}{\text{Hb\%/dl of the transfused blood}}$$

Whole blood, 10–13 g/dl; packed cells, 18–23 g/dl.
Blood volume is approximately equal to 70–80 ml/kg body weight.
Because anaemia is so common and the estimation of Hb so simple, no anaesthetic should be given before a Hb result is available. If this is low by

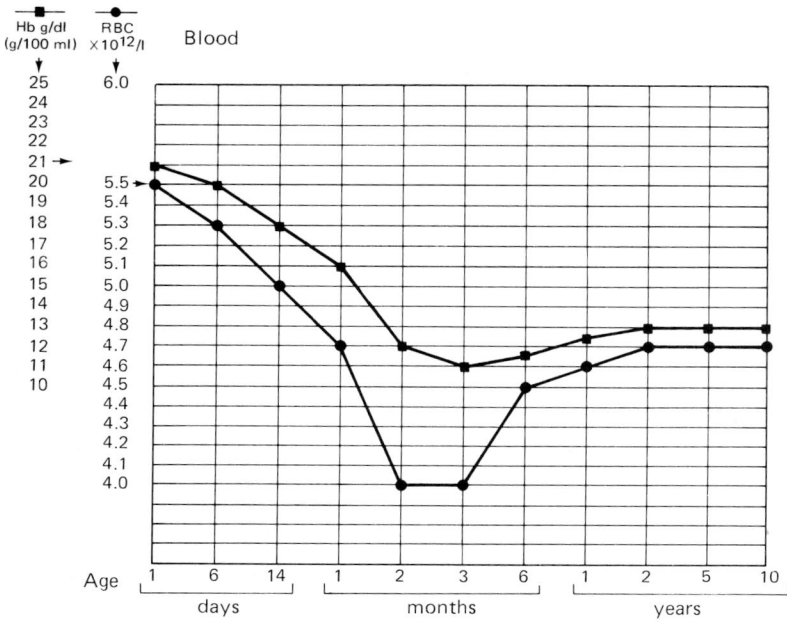

Fig. 4.1 Normal variation of haemoglobin concentration with age.

the standards of the local laboratory, then the cause should be ascertained and treated, if time permits (Fig. 4.1).

Though a lower limit of *10 g/dl* is a useful working guide, there is no general agreement as to what level of Hb carries an increased risk for anaesthesia. The low levels of Hb seen in paediatric patients can be compensated for by increased red cell 2,3-DPG, which allows increased oxygen delivery to the tissues and a lower erythropoietin drive, and hence a lower red cell mass. The increased organic phosphates are secondary to the increase in inorganic phosphates seen in these patients.

The decision to operate or not can only be made when all facets of the situation (e.g. urgency of the surgery) have been considered.

Red cell 2,3-DPG and oxygen affinity

There exists within the red cell a mechanism which allows control of the oxygen affinity of the Hb and depends on the interaction of Hb with organic phosphates within the cell. Eighty per cent of the active phosphate is 2,3-DPG.

2,3-DPG binds specifically to deoxyhaemoglobin and thereby stabilizes the deoxy form of Hb and allows less oxygen affinity in this state. The central cavity of relaxed oxyhaemoglobin is smaller and is thus unable to accommodate 2,3-DPG.

When intracellular 2,3-DPG increases, tissue oxygenation improves as the

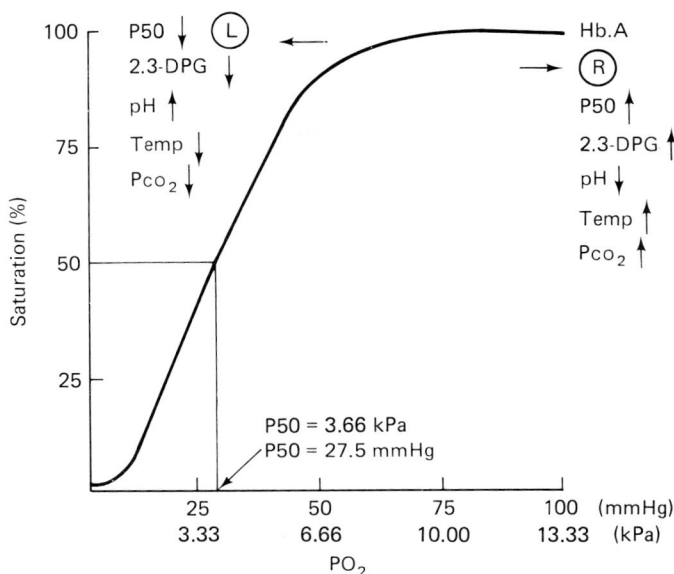

Fig. 4.2   Factors controlling the position of the oxygen dissociation curve.

oxygen dissociation curve is shifted to the right and the P50 is increased. (The P50 is the partial pressure of oxygen when the Hb is 50 per cent saturated and is increased by a fall in the Hb (Bohr effect).) This fall in Hb also causes a decrease in 2,3-DPG. Fig. 4.2 illustrates the factors controlling the position of the oxygen dissociation curve. The pH effect on the oxygen dissociation curve is seen at once whereas the effect of the falling 2,3-DPG level takes several hours to develop. Thus 2,3-DPG can affect the oxygen affinity, not only by a direct effect on P50 but also by control of the pH within the red cell. It is thought that about 35 per cent of the change in oxygen affinity caused by alteration in 2,3-DPG levels may be explained by the effect of 2,3-DPG on the red cell pH. There is an increase in 2,3-DPG with cardiac failure, an effect which parallels the fall in cardiac output. In congenital heart disease, an increase is seen when the mean Pa_{O_2} falls to below 8 kPa (60 mmHg). Increases are also part of the physiological adaptation to altitude—the alkalosis secondary to hypoxic-induced hyperventilation stimulates the increased 2,3-DPG levels.

Shifts to the right of the oxygen dissociation curve are of great advantage to the anaemic patient and is one of the reasons why patients with chronic renal failure on maintenance dialysis can survive with low Hb. Those patients with chronic renal failure but not on dialysis do not have an increased 2,3-DPG level, but this may possibly be prevented by an accompanying acidosis.

Stored blood for transfusion

Valtis and Kennedy (1954) first showed that the oxygen dissociation curve of stored blood is shifted to the left and that a large fall in 2,3-DPG levels occurs during the first 15 days of storage. The levels are much better preserved in citrate phosphate dextrose (CPD) than in acid citrate dextrose (ACD) blood. After transfusion, the levels of 2,3-DPG in donor cells is restored within the recipient, though this is not an immediate process and must depend on the volume of stored blood and its age. The rate of restoration also depends on the cardiorespiratory function and the acid–base status of the recipient, and is probably not complete within 24 hours.

As already discussed, there is a compensatory mechanism for the decrease in oxygen flux seen with a chronic anaemia. The increase in the ability of the red cells to unload oxygen in the tissues under the influence of a raised 2,3-DPG level may be seriously disrupted by an ACD blood transfusion. If preoperative blood transfusion is thought to be necessary, it should be carried out at least 48 hours before surgery, using fresh CPD blood. In this way it is possible to achieve acceptable levels of both Hb and 2,3-DPG. After massive blood transfusion and the exchange transfusion associated with cardiopulmonary bypass, the 2,3-DPG levels are not normal again for up to three days (Macdonald, 1977).

During pregnancy, the 2,3-DPG rises by about 20 per cent thus maintaining normal maternal tissue oxygenation and benefiting the baby with its high-affinity Hb F. Hb F itself does not interact with 2,3-DPG, which explains the very high oxygen affinity of this Hb. Because of this, an ACD transfusion would be dangerous for the baby.

Haemoglobinopathies and sickling

More than 100 haemoglobinopathies have been detected; in most cases abnormal molecular structure can be directly related to disordered function and to the production of clinical manifestations.

The normal adult Hb (Hb.A) has four polypeptide chains: two α chains each with 141 amino acid residues and two β chains with 146 residues, whereas Hb.F consists of α_2 and γ_2. Each chain has a haem group and an iron atom to each chain.

A separate gene determines the amino acid sequences of each chain.

If the stereochemical relationships are disturbed, oxygen binding may be abnormal or there may be other deleterious effects on the Hb molecule.

A single amino acid substitution in one type of polypeptide chain is accounted for by replacement of one nucleotide in an RNA code. It takes only a change in a single purine in the codon which specifies the sixth amino acid of the β chain so that glutamic acid replaces valine, to give the abnormal sickle Hb.S.

Thalassaemia is the inherited impairment of Hb synthesis caused by retarded production of a specific type of globin chain and is not associated with a primary structural abnormality.

All haemoglobinopathies are inherited as autosomal codominant traits and the heterozygote will have both normal and abnormal Hb in each cell, though the normal will predominate. The genes which determine the structure of one class of globin chains are alleles; i.e. a person heterozygous for Hb.S and Hb.C (both abnormalities in the β chain) has no Hb.A and transmits one or other, not both, to each child. All occur because of mutations. Hb.S seems to protect infants against the lethal falciparum malaria, which probably accounts for the maintenance of this deleterious abnormality in Africa.

Most haemoglobinopathies have been discovered by abnormal electrophoretic mobility, though some have the same pattern using standard techniques.

Sickle cell disease

Sickle cell disease was first described by J. B. Herrick in 1910, and in 1927 Hahn and Gillespie showed that the distortion of the red cell is related to the state of oxygenation of the Hb. From his discovery in 1949 of the abnormal Hb, Pauling (1953) developed the concept of 'disease at the molecular level'.

The condition is caused by a single amino acid substitution in the β chain. There is no effect on oxygen affinity but there is a unique intermolecular reaction in which molecules of deoxygenated Hb.S tend to form insoluble aggregates (tactoids) which distort the erythrocyte and increase its rigidity—the so-called process of sickling. The attractive forces between molecules operate only over short distances, so sickling is influenced only by the concentration of desaturated Hb in the cell. Conditions affecting oxygen desaturation and the pH in the cell are critical to the degree of sickling—as is the presence of another Hb, which may interact with Hb.S to lessen or enhance sickling. Except for a few irreversible sickled cells, the red cells resume their shape when reoxygenated.

Sickle cell disease is the clinical expression of the homozygous state of Hb.S. Because of intravascular trapping in small vessels and increased destruction in the reticuloendothelial system, the clinical picture is one of unrelenting haemolytic anaemia (5–8 g/dl). In addition, there are recurrent attacks of pain and fever as many organs (e.g. spleen) become involved in episodes of infarction.

Among Negroes in West Africa the incidence of homozygous sickle cell disease is 1–2 per cent (20–30 per cent trait). Eighty per cent die before the age of 2 years. In the USA, where 16 in 10 000 are calculated to be homozygous at conception, the condition is not as severe. This is possibly because general medical care, control of crisis-provoking infections and treatment of chronic anaemias may be better. Apart from pregnancy and the postpartum period, the condition tends to be less severe in adult life.

Sickle cell trait

Carriers of this condition (the heterozygous form) are found in the popula
tions of Africa, the Mediterranean (two surveys in Greece show an incidence
of 26·9 and 20·6 per cent), the Middle East and India. The concentration
of Hb.S is usually low (20–50 per cent) so that no sickling occurs at physiological levels of Po$_2$. However, sickling may occur and infarction of the spleen
is a risk if these people fly in unpressurized aircraft. Sickling has been described in cases of cyanotic congenital heart disease and also associated with
general anaesthesia. The organs at particular risk in the sickle trait patient
appear to be the spleen and kidneys. Sickling may occur in the sluggish,
poorly organized perfusion in the spleen and in the renal medulla where
oxygen tension, pH and tonicity are all conducive to sickling. Renal disorders, including haematuria and renal papillary necrosis, are all more common in individuals with sickle cell trait than in the general population (Leading article, 1976).

The combinations of Hb.S with other abnormal haemoglobins occur. The
most important of these is Hb.SC, which occurs at one-quarter of the frequency of sickle cell disease in the USA; it is characterized by a mild anaemia,
an enlarged spleen and the occurrence of vascular occlusions and bone
necroses.

Other similar conditions occur with Hb.F and with the combination of
Hb.S and thalassaemia, but these are less common.

The crises which arise with sickle cell disease can be classified into two
groups: haematological and painful.

(1) *Haematological* crises occur in three ways:

(a) *Sequestration* crises ensue when there is a sudden great increase in
the number of sickled red cells, often provoked by hypoxia, venous desaturation, acidaemia, etc. The cells become trapped in the spleen and by other
cells of the reticuloendothelial system, causing a severe and occasionally
fatal deficiency of circulating red cells.

(b) *Haemolytic* crises occur with a more gradual sickling process.

(c) *Aplastic* crises occur for reasons not fully understood (though perhaps related to deficiency of folic acid) and in which the bone marrow
enters an aplastic phase. As the red cells have a much shortened life anyway, and erythropoiesis has ceased, the Hb will rapidly fall to a very low
and even fatal level.

(2) *Painful* crises are the clinical manifestation of the sickling process and
its results.

As sickling occurs, blood viscosity increases which leads to increased stasis
and a vicious cycle of sickling is established. The red blood cell debris can
cause painful vascular occlusions in bones, and particularly in the spleen.
The abdominal pain of a painful sickle crisis may mimic the 'acute abdomen'
in which pain, tenderness and 'rebound' are seen. Intracerebral infarction
with neurological damage is also a common sequel to an episode of this type.
The factors which can provoke a crisis in sickle cell disease include general
anaesthesia (in which hypoxia, acidaemia, hypothermia and vascular stasis

are all a possibility), hypermetabolic states (febrile illnesses and thyrotoxicosis) and hypoxic illnesses (pneumonia). With Hb.SA and Hb.SC the position is less clear though there are reports of splenic infarcts and haematuria following anaesthesia and flights in aircraft. The combination of Hb.S and Hb.C seems to be a particularly hazardous one. Sudden and severe sickling crises and splenic infarction can occur—especially associated with general anaesthesia.

Huntsman, Green and Serjeant (1971) describe seven cases of sickling crises provoked by flight in aircraft and claim that only patients with complicated sickle trait will sickle in these circumstances. However, Jones, Binder and Donowho (1970) describe four fatal cases following moderate exercise at an altitude of 1234 m (1345 ft). It would appear that Hb.SA is not a risk in normal aircraft which are pressurized to 2600–3300 m (8000–10 000 ft) equivalent, but that it could become a risk with high flying in an unpressurized light plane. Carriers of Hb.SC probably should not use air transport. It is for this reason that all aircrew should be screened for abnormal Hb, and if it is accepted that anaesthesia presents similar risk, all patients who are at risk of carrying the trait should be screened as well. This should now be standard practice in all hospitals.

The detection of Hb.S in the laboratory depends on the abnormal physical properties of this particular Hb molecule (Leading article, 1972).

(1) Electrophoresis reflects the net positive charge on the molecule because of the replacement of valine by glutamic acid. This technique can detect concentrations of Hb.S as low as 5 per cent—e.g. the concentration in umbilical cord blood or after transfusion of normal patients with sickle blood. Hb.D and Hb.G have similar mobility and can give false positive readings. These tests take 24–48 hours but are vital for complete diagnosis.

(2) A sickling test depends on the distortion of the red cell membrane associated with linear polymerization of Hb.S molecules when deoxygenated. The blood is incubated with a powerful reducing agent (2 per cent sodium metabisulphite solution) on a microscope slide. The rate of sickling is proportional to the concentration of Hb.S. Sickling is specific to the $\beta6$ valine substitution which is confined to Hb.S and the much rarer Hb.C(Harlem).

(3) Solubility tests depend on the fact that deoxygenated Hb.S is relatively insoluble in phosphate buffers of high molar concentration. These are suitable for automation, are rapid, reliable, simple and cheap, and there is an obvious end point to read. The proprietary Sickledex detects Hb.S by precipitation. It is simple and reliable, and good for emergencies though expensive for widespread screening programmes.

A screening sickle test should be performed for all patients at risk of carrying sickle cell disease. Where positive, electrophoresis must be set up. These are most conveniently started when the patient is first put on the surgical waiting list, or in an anaesthetic clinic. In an emergency a patient with a positive sickle test should be treated as if the electrophoresis showed homozygous sickle cell disease. The level of Hb can be helpful because a patient with an Hb of 12 g/dl or more is unlikely to have Hb.SS, though patients with Hb.SC usually also have a normal Hb level.

The anaesthetic management of all cases requires great care and attention to detail (Howells *et al.*, 1972). Where possible, any anaemia must be treated preoperatively; Brown (1965) accepts the Hb above 8 g/dl though other authors prefer it to be above 10 g/dl in children. For elective surgery, a time of minimal haemolysis and maximum erythropoiesis should be chosen. Transfusion carries an increased risk of adverse reactions and over-transfusion will increase the viscosity of the blood without necessarily diluting the cells carrying Hb.S. This, theoretically at least, will increase the risk of vascular occlusion. It is also known that the oxygen dissociation curve is shifted to the right (more oxygen is given up in the tissues) to compensate for the anaemia, and if 2,3-DPG-deficient blood is transfused the curve will move to the left and tissue oxygenation may suffer (Lenfant, Bellingham and Detter, 1972). Partial exchange transfusion is the most satisfactory treatment and is effective in preventing crises when 50 per cent of the sickle cells have been replaced by normal cells; 11 ml/kg body weight of packed cells can be transfused every 12 hours until the Hb is 14 g/dl. After four days, about 50 per cent will have been exchanged. After ten days with reduced marrow function, nearly all the sickle cells will have been destroyed. Folic acid prophylaxis is usually given to the carriers of Hb.SS and Hb.SC. Possibly a more satisfactory method, where time allows, is to give two transfusions of fresh CPD blood: one three weeks and the other three days before surgery is to take place. The aim is to achieve a Hb of approximately 12 g/dl and an electrophoresis which shows a percentage of Hb.S within the range seen in heterozygous patients. Surgery and anaesthesia will therefore carry lower risks. If the last transfusion is given three days before surgery, the red cell levels of 2,3-DPG should be normal.

It is essential to eliminate infections. Febrile episodes can lead to crises and *Salmonella* is especially liable to be pathogenic. Severe pulmonary infections with respiratory distress and hypoxia can cause a crisis even with Hb.SA.

Conduct of anaesthesia in general terms should seek to avoid those factors which are known to be responsible for the sickling process: hypoxia, acidaemia, vascular stasis and hypothermia.

Hypoxia is always the basic cause of a sickle cell crisis, so low inspired oxygen concentrations and respiratory depression are to be avoided. Non-respiratory depressant premedication is recommended and standard induction agents are safe. At least 30 per cent oxygen is needed to maintain a normal Pa_{O_2} during anaesthesia, but 50 per cent oxygen with nitrous oxide will allow a safety margin. Respiratory depression, respiratory obstruction and laryngeal spasm must be avoided. Provided these conditions are met, there is no contraindication to any particular anaesthetic technique.

Measures should be taken to minimize stasis during surgery. Tourniquets, theoretically harmful, seem to be no problem with careful exsanguination, but probably should not be used where Hb.SS and Hb.SC are present. Thoracic anaesthesia is safe with Hb.SA provided great care is taken to avoid perioperative hypoxaemia (Searle, 1972).

During surgical operations the temperature in the superficial leg veins may fall to 30°C. At this temperature, blood is 30 per cent more viscous than at 37°C. Thus patients should be kept warm at all times to prevent this fall in peripheral temperature and steps taken to prevent peripheral vasoconstriction.

Alkalosis has been shown to give an increased resistance to hypoxia of the red cells, and many workers favour an alkali regimen for patients with Hb. SS about to undergo surgery (Greenberg and Kass, 1958). Sodium bicarbonate 0·5–1·0 g/kg body weight per day orally will keep the urine alkaline. This may be given for two days preoperatively. Alternatively, 3·3 mEq/kg sodium bicarbonate solution intravenously in one hour will keep the urine alkaline for 6–12 hours.

2,3-DPG and sickling

The induction of metabolic alkalosis using sodium bicarbonate increases the oxygen affinity of Hb and decreases the likelihood of sickling. When bicarbonate is given orally, there is time for the pH change to increase 2,3-DPG and counteract the pH effect on the oxygen dissociation curve, and in this case no benefit would be achieved; however, intravenous bicarbonate would tide the patient over the peroperative and immediate postoperative periods without causing changes in 2,3-DPG.

An increased inspired oxygen concentration should be administered by suitable means (headbox, controlled-concentration facemask such as the Venturi mask, nasal prongs, etc.) in the postoperative period. This will prevent the postoperative hypoxia frequently seen after thoracic and abdominal surgery, and will cover the period during which it may be necessary to give respiratory-depressant analgesic drugs. Oxygen therapy for longer than 24 hours is unnecessary and may cause further depression of the output of the bone marrow. Oduro and Searle (1972) suggest that alkalinization is unnecessary if a simple and safe anaesthetic technique is used.

Occlusive crises

The treatment for occlusive crises when they occur consists of analgesia, vasodilators and blood transfusion if the Hb falls below 5 g/dl. Alkalinization does not relieve the crisis once it is occurring. Dextran 40 has been advocated as a useful agent to increase peripheral blood flow and to mobilize trapped cells, but reports of success are conflicting. Watson-Williams (1963) described three cases where pain was reduced or cured, but Reidenberg and Barry (1964) had two cases where dextran 40 had no obvious effect and caused sensitivity in one patient who received it twice.

Others have suggested the use of phenothiazines which may suppress the reduction of Hb.S; of magnesium sulphate which prevents the formation of a permanent thrombus and may mobilize sludged erythrocytes; or urea in an osmotically balanced invert sugar solution which can inhibit and reverse sickling in both homo- and heterozygous intact red cells *in vitro* (this has not been confirmed).

Regular transfusion therapy can maintain elevated Hb concentration and keep the concentration of Hb.S down as low as 30 per cent. This has been shown to prevent progressive cerebrovascular changes where these were occurring in a particular patient (Russell *et al.*, 1976).

References

Brain, M. C. (1975). The anemias. In: *Textbook of Medicine*. Ed. by P. B. Beeson. W. B. Saunders, Philadelphia.

Brown, R. A. (1965). Anaesthesia in patients with sickle cell anaemia. *British Journal of Anaesthesia* **37**, 181.

Cullen, D. J. and Eger, E. I. (1970). The effects of hypoxia and isovolemic anemia on the halothane requirements (MAC) of dogs. III. The effects of acute isovolemic anemia. *Anesthesiology* **32**, 46.

Gillies, I. D. S. (1974). Anaemia and anaesthesia. *British Journal of Anaesthesia* **46**, 589.

Greenberg, M. S. and Kass, E. H. (1958). Studies on the destruction of red blood cells. XIII. Observations on the role of pH in the pathogenesis and treatment of painful crises in sickle cell disease. *Archives of Internal Medicine* **101**, 355.

Hahn, E. V. and Gillespie, E. B. (1927). Sickle cell anaemia: report of cases, greatly improved by splenectomy. Experimental study of sickle cell formation. *Archives of Internal Medicine* **39**, 233.

Herrick, J. B. (1910). Peculiar elongated and sickle shape red blood corpuscles in a case of severe anaemia. *Archives of Internal Medicine* **6**, 517.

Howells, T. H., Huntsman, R. G., Boys, J. E. and Mahmood, A. (1972). Anaesthesia and sickle cell haemoglobin. *British Journal of Anaesthesia* **44**, 975.

Huntsman, R. G., Green, R. L. and Serjeant, G. R. (1971). The sickle cell and altitude. *British Medical Journal* **4**, 593.

Jones, S. R., Binder, R. A. and Donowho, E. M. (1970). Sudden death in sickle cell trait. *New England Journal of Medicine* **282**, 323.

Leading article (1972). Detecting sickle haemoglobin. *British Medical Journal* **2**, 246.

Leading article (1976). Sickle cell trait. *British Medical Journal* **1**, 1359.

Lenfant, C., Bellingham, A. J. and Detter, J. C. (1972). Physiological factors influencing the haemoglobin affinity for oxygen. In: *Oxygen Affinity of Haemoglobin and Red Cell Acid Base Status*, 4th Alfred Benyon Symposium, Copenhagen, 1971, p. 736. Munksgaard, Copenhagen.

Macdonald, R. (1977). Red cell 2,3-diphosphoglycerate and oxygen affinity. *Anaesthesia* **32**, 544.

Nunn, J. F. (1969). *Applied Respiratory Physiology*. Butterworths, London.

Oduro, K. A. and Searle, J. F. (1972). Anaesthesia in sickle cell states: a plea for simplicity. *British Medical Journal* **4**, 596.

Pauling, L. (1953). Abnormality of hemogloblin molecule in hereditary hemolytic anemia. *Harvey Lectures*, 1953–1954, p. 216.

Reidenberg, M. and Barry, W. E. (1964). Low molecular weight dextran. *Lancet* **i**, 988.

Russell, M. O., Goldberg, H. I., Reis, L., Friedman, S., Slater, R., Reivich, M. and Schwartz, E. (1976). Transfusion therapy for cerebrovascular abnormality in sickle cell disease. *Journal of Pediatrics* **88**, 382.

Searle, J. F. (1972). Anaesthesia and sickle cell haemoglobin. *British Journal of Anaesthesia* **44**, 1335.

Valtis, D. J. and Kennedy, A. C. (1954). Defective gas-transport function of stored red blood cells. *Lancet* **i**, 119.

Watson-Williams, E. J. (1963). Sickle cell crisis treated with rheomacrodex. *Lancet* **i**, 1053.

Index